THE YOGA MENTOR

Celest Pereira

Published by **Celest Pereira** 2016

First published in Great Britain in 2016

by **Celest Pereira**

Table of Contents

DEDICATION

To the yoga teachers of this world.
I admire you all!

About the Author

If you've picked this book up my guess is that you've just finished your yoga teacher training and you are a little unsure of how to get started on your teaching career. It's scary going from the safe haven of the training into a classroom full of people that expect you to lead. How do you even get a group of people to agree to come to your class? Or what centre will hire you with no experience to teach for them?

There are many unknowns when you start. My calling to write this book was born out of the desire to see other yoga teachers flourishing in their careers. A lot of newly qualified teachers take endless courses, one after the other, while doing a job they tolerate, in the hope that one day they will be able to leave their job and follow their heart's calling: to teach yoga for a living. I know this because many newly-qualified teachers often come to me for advice on how to get started with their careers.

But why? Who am I? Let me introduce myself. My name is Celest Pereira, a yoga teacher from London. It's so nice to meet you my fellow yoga teacher. Thank you for picking this book and reading it. I am not writing a book that is the industry standard on how to become a successful yoga teacher. But rather, this book is a chance for me to share my own personal story on what I did to live a life of abundance teaching yoga. I want you to get to where I am in half the time it took me, and then surpass my level (if that is your dream). I want this book to cut your learning time so if you want to make yoga your livelihood, you will without a doubt find a way! I'm by no means a 'finished product'. If anything I am still learning and making many mistakes. But what I have learnt I want you to know too, so we can all grow together.

My teaching career began because I was trying to break into the health industry as a physiotherapist. While applying for jobs, I taught a few yoga classes on the side to earn money and before I knew it, my passion for teaching was ignited and morphed into a sense of fulfilment that was too good to give up. That was only a few years ago and nowadays I'm teaching in top studios in London; have been flown to exotic locations to teach clients; am an ambassador for international brands; have been featured in advertising campaigns; have published articles; am running sold-out retreats; am teaching at international yoga festivals; and have created an online platform that allows me to earn a passive income through my online teaching downloads.

This didn't happen because I'm extremely clever, gifted or special. On the contrary, I make mistakes all the time. I say stupid things, fart, trip and fall over. I am as human as they come. I am also dyslexic and even found writing my own name a struggle when I was at school! Everything I did took twice as much time and work than it did my peers to get the same results. The positive flip side of my dyslexia is that from a young age I learned that no matter what the obstacle, hard work pays off.

My academic struggles fed my love of movement and dance. Dancing was the one activity that fed my confidence and made me feel like I was capable of being great at something. I wasn't a gifted dancer but it was my passion. And that, I believed, was enough. Unfortunately, along with challenging your ability to read and write, dyslexia messes with your ability to process information quickly. Consequently, I couldn't pick up routines quickly enough in auditions to get any dance jobs. So I completed a few courses and became a qualified gym instructor instead. Earning £12,000 a year, the lowest rung on the money food chain.

Needless to say, I had drifted quite far from my passion of being a professional dancer and was feeling very despondent and unfulfilled. Noticing my enthusiasm wane, one or two people gave me advice and encouraged me to go to university to study. Other than dance, my only other interest lay in physiotherapy. However, becoming a physio would mean embarking on a Bachelor of Science degree and I thought this career path was way out of my academic league. I mean, hello… I didn't even finish school.

Despite my reservations, I applied and got into the programme and four years later surprised myself by passing all my exams with good grades. Like my younger school days, I had to work twice as hard as everyone else and found the course extremely challenging. There were a few meltdowns and many tears. But the struggle was definitely worth it. I walked away from that degree with a piece of paper that not only qualified me to practice physiotherapy, but also with the belief that nothing is impossible!

Yoga came into my life before this tiny detour, when I was at dance college at the tender age of 17. Early on a Wednesday morning a tall, dreamy silver fox would come and deliver yoga classes to the dancers. I was amazed at how difficult I found the balance aspects of the practice. I thought I would be a total bad ass at yoga, given my dance background. I could not have been more wrong. It was a challenge that I found very stimulating. I drifted away from yoga for a short while, but life has a funny habit of pointing you in certain directions. One such daily signpost was when I walked passed a yoga studio and saw an Ashtanga yoga class being taught, and I was taken aback by the beauty and symmetry of the human body. Then I actually stepped inside and tried the class and my mental dialogue became, "OMG! I forgot how hard it is to pretzel your body on one leg whilst looking zen."

As I mentioned earlier, I decided to explore the idea of going to university. But I also began to love the idea of deepening my yoga practice and learning more about the philosophical aspects of yoga. So I began researching teacher trainings. I spent hours on Google looking up various schools. In the end I was sold on one thing: price! (Not the best reason to buy or invest). I had so little money I had to go somewhere that wouldn't cost much. But, I was also desperate to do an Ashtanga yoga course. God forbid I should do anything Hatha based (yawn!) I look back and I have to laugh at the irony. I found a school in India that was exactly in my price range. For £500 I had a full month of teacher training, all my accommodation and food costs covered, along with any books and learning materials. Result! I was thrilled. However little did I know, that this Indian school was using the words, Ashtanga yoga in Google analytics to refer to Patanjali's eight limbs of yoga and not the set sequence laid out by Pattabhi Jois. This school was the most classical, Hatha based yoga course under the sun.

I arrived a little shocked and maybe even slightly annoyed. "Great" I thought, "a whole month of slow boring yoga" (Could I have had a worse attitude?). Thankfully that month ended up being the best month of my life. The course taught us the ancient practices of yoga, such as the cleansing rituals, chanting, meditation and karma yoga. We had to drink salt water and vomit it out; use a netti pot to rinse water through our nasal cavities; we woke up at 4am daily to start the morning practice; and we had no coffee, tea, meat or alcohol at all. This might sound like torture. I certainly thought it was for the first week. But then things started to shift for me. I started to walk slowly again, I noticed the colours of nature around me and I took time to appreciate every bite of food. That month taught me in quite a literal sense what Ghandi had said, "there is more to life than increasing its speed." All of these seemingly strange practices I think added to what I call my yoga super powers (my ability to make others feel good).

I was buzzing after India but as soon as I returned to the UK I was hit with a challenge. The physiotherapy market was flooded with newly qualified post-graduates, making competition fierce and jobs scarce. I applied for numerous jobs but couldn't land a solid, full-time position that was near to where I lived. It was here that my journey as a yoga teacher began.

Out of pure desperation, I started teaching yoga to earn survival money. Ironically, this career 'diversion' led me to my real calling. As French poet, Jean de La Fontaine once said, "A person often meets his destiny on the road he took to avoid it." This was true for me. I very quickly I realised that teaching yoga made me happier than anything else and that this 'side job' could become a fulfilling and sustainable livelihood. I felt like I was honing all the superpowers I'd developed in India, reading books and meditating. I loved how sharing what I knew made a difference to the people in my class.

I learnt a lot of lessons during my transition from teacher-in-training to yoga entrepreneur. This book contains everything I wish I knew before I started teaching. I've divided the information and first-hand advice into six categories. Along with my own insights, I have included personal anecdotes and helpful advice from other successful teachers I've met along the way.

Embark covers how to get started. How to gain classes and clients and how to earn money doing what you love.

Elevate covers how to take what you're doing to the next level so that it's sustainable. This section reveals steps to take to make teaching an abundant resource and includes information about hosting workshops and retreats.

Expert delves into the concept of becoming an expert in your field and covers ways to become known in your community as the 'go-to person' for your particular yoga style. It outlines various tips and techniques to expand your professional profile, how to build a loyal student following, and how to build a sustainable, long-term career.

Economics shows you how to make ends meet as a teacher and includes budgeting and investment tips.

Energy tells you why your health is so pivotal in helping you excel in your yoga teaching career and outlines simple strategies for maintaining good health.

Evolve reveals personal development tools that have positively supported and transformed my career and life.

My ultimate goal with this book is to get you to the highest level you choose to go, locally or internationally.

Either way, I want you to become known as a superhero within your community! To get to the point where you can use all the great skills you've picked up in your life and teacher training to enhance peoples lives and be the best teacher you can possibly be. To get you there I will share everything I did every step of the way.

The great decisions I made along with all the stupid mistakes. So my new friend and superhero in-the-making, roll out your mat, take a deep breath, and let's begin.

Chapter 1

EMBARK

The Downward Dog of Your Teaching Career

Remember the very first time you ever did a downward dog? Remember how painful it was? How your arms felt like they might collapse and your legs could just snap? Remember how happy you were when the teacher told you to start cycling through your legs as that eased some of your discomfort? Well superhero, that cycle through your legs is what I'm going to teach you now. But don't be fooled. It's still going to be uncomfortable. And yes, you will have to to get comfortable with the uncomfortable!

Take uncomfortable Sarah, a newly qualified yoga teacher hoping to break into the world of teaching. "I'm so scared! I can't imagine teaching a class, Celest. I feel a panicking sensation when I think of getting up in front of all those people. What if someone asks me something I don't know? What if I say the wrong name of a pose!" I wanted to tell Sarah that when she started teaching some magical force would overcome her and she would transform into a brilliant teacher and that insecure feelings would vanish. But that would be a lie. The truth is, I too suffered from this concern when I first started teaching and was terrified that someone in the class was going to ask me what the Sanskrit name of every pose was, or which specific muscles were being used.

Many teachers who approach me for guidance about how to get started have one major fear in common: the fear of not knowing enough. This fear is what makes most teachers doubt themselves and enroll in course after course, in the hope that they'll discover the secret to becoming a successful teacher. In my case, my saving grace was that I didn't have any choice. I needed to pay my bills and had no other option than to feel the fear and do it anyway. This taught me two important things:

99.99% of the people that come to your classes will be humble, lovely and want to get the most out of the class. In all my years of teaching, I've only had one or two students ask me the Sanskrit name of a certain pose during a class. Few, if any, will challenge you in front of everyone else, and if they do then that experience will only help you grow as a teacher and a leader. I also learned that there is no shame in admitting what you don't know. When someone asks me a question that I can't answer, I confidently tell the person in front of the entire class that I don't know the answer to their question. I then open the question out to everyone in the room. Many times people in the class have been practicing for a very long time. So they have a lot of knowledge. I love asking the class questions. To do this is a sign of a teacher that does not put themselves above their students. I still firmly believe that no student is less than his or her teacher and no teacher is above his or her students either. So when confronted with questions that put your knowledge under question, please don't worry. You are a human being that is doing your best. Admitting that is a beautiful thing.

No course will automatically turn you into a good teacher, only practice can do that. *Nothing* can replace experience. Start your career by accepting that you might not be an outstanding teacher right away. In fact, expect to teach many classes that aren't great and learn, learn, learn! I'm still learning every day and even after all these years, sometimes teach classes that aren't amazing. These 'terrible' classes used to happen to me all the time, now they are less frequent. Had I not been through the messy classes that left me cringing and wishing the earth would swallow me whole, I wouldn't have transcended to new levels. The best advice I can give is…get used to being crap. Because you're going to teach hundreds of rubbish classes. And each and every one that you teach is necessary. Without these terrible classes you won't progress and transform. You can only get better through practice, so leave your ego at the door and walk into each class with humility (not fear!).

How to Start Teaching
Gyms & Community Centres

One of the best places to start your career as a yoga teacher is within gyms and community centres. The clientele in these centres are usually interested in a variety of activities. Hence, yoga is either something new that they have added to their activities list, or something they wish to use to enhance the other activities they partake in. Less frequently will the hard core yogi be in these centres seeking to deepen their practice, and that's what makes it such great training ground.

You see the hardcore yogi might not be your ideal client

just yet (more about that later), but if you want to teach in top yoga centres, this is the person who you will have to appeal to eventually. Still, don't be fooled. Gone are the days that you can just waltz into a gym or community centre with your CV and hope they will call you. In cities like London, to get into these centres you need to connect with the right people and off the back of that, become the best cover teacher these lovely gym loving/ yogi people have ever met in their entire lives! How to you become a great cover teacher? Let's look at that next.

Cover Teaching

Ok so now for the big question: how do you start gaining real experience in real yoga gyms and community centres? As I said before, the first thing to do is to become a cover teacher. This is an essential stepping-stone and a vital step into taking off your yoga teaching 'trainer wheels'. Don't expect to walk into top yoga centres (or anywhere for that matter) and be given work immediately. The old fashioned method of walking into a venue with a CV in hand and a big smile unfortunately sends the message that you are just getting started, have no experience, and are perhaps a bit desperate. Ouch! I know how harsh that sounds but that is what I have personally heard people who own centres say. To be fair, this might be my narrow perspective living in a busy city like London. In other parts of the world it might be much easier.

But let's just assume in this book, nothing comes easy. That way, no surprises will take you off guard. I want you to be ready for anything!

Support Other Superhero's

To become a cover teacher, you need to find teachers whose classes you love, and support them sincerely. Build a relationship with other superhero's in your community and tell them that you would love to be on their 'emergency cover list'. Why is this wording appropriate? Because many teachers already have a list of favourite backup teachers to turn to when planning their holiday covers. However, what happens to every teacher (and this will no doubt happen to you too) is last minute emergencies.

When these come up teachers will frantically call every teacher in their phone book. If you have told the teacher you are happy to take on any emergency covers, there is a good chance the teacher will get in touch with you before anyone else. It's very important that when this happens you drop everything to go and teach the class. Of course, if you still have a full-time job, don't get fired for walking out the door; but if you just need to adjust your social schedule, do it. If you don't like letting people down, you can even consider telling everyone that they shouldn't take it personally if you cancel on them last minute for a six-month period. Be honest and tell them about your ambition to become a yoga teacher and that you are determined to get on a few cover lists. True friends will understand and it'll be worth it.

In my experience, most of my cover work has come from teachers that I've supported and built a relationship with. By 'supported' I mean I've attended their classes, workshops and events, so have witnessed and experienced their teaching style first-hand and therefore knew what their loyal clients enjoyed (in terms of the style and intensity). More than that, I had made an effort to get to know the teachers personally. I wasn't a faceless name on an email asking for cover or classes. I was a real person that made an effort. Consequently, if they needed a cover teacher, they'd pass the class to me.

Once you have covered a few classes, the next step is to ask if you can be considered for regular cover teaching. Also, make it clear to these amazing, supportive teachers that you are happy to take on any cover they are offered that they might not want. As my career grew I would get offered loads of classes to cover that I had no time to teach. If someone told me they wanted more work, I would simply forward them the email time and time again, till I could see they were good to step out on their own. Please, however, don't be a nag. I always go out of my way to help newly qualified teachers, but if they bombard me with nagging messages I tend to take a step back. I also tend to avoid the teachers who are overly negative. My energy is precious, I give a lot when I am teaching, and negative people make me tired. So if you feel negative or don't have anything good to say, be aware of your impact on the person you are meeting up with. There is one teacher that regularly asked me to sit with her and give advice. But the time we had together she would moan and complain the whole time.In the end I started to avoid contact with her, because I didn't feel it was serving either of us spending time together.

Get to Know the Class Coordinators

Make a point of asking if there is any way that you can help support the studio's class coordinator. Scheduled classes are constantly changing in any studio and the goal is to be the first person in the coordinator's mind when they're shuffling classes and looking for a replacement teacher. Think about it, if you were a coordinator and had to create a new class on the schedule, would you ask someone who has spoken to you in person, told you they've had great feedback from members, and made an effort to ask how they could support the studio? Or would you randomly pick from the long list of faceless names on a database? Again the key here is patience. This process takes time and sincerity. Trust that the more you put yourself out there the better and easier it will become to eventually make the crossover between cover teacher and having a regular slot of your own.

Master Your 'Teaching Voice'

Once you manage to land a regular teaching gig, the next hurdle to overcome is your (possible) lack of experience in leading a group of people – something that is extremely intimidating when you're just starting out. My recommendation is to create a supportive environment where you can practice using your 'teaching voice' – which is really your voice but a tiny bit louder and more commanding. Enlist help from people who are supportive of your goal to become a teacher and ask them if they're interested in taking some free yoga classes with you to help you build your confidence. Make it very clear that after a few months the 'free' aspect will have to change, so that there is no misunderstanding.

Special Note:

On the topic of a 'teaching voice'. I am not keen on the 'yoga voice'. Do you know what I mean? The one that's all breathy and holy and (cough) - sorry that was me choking on a small amount of vomit. Personally there is a serious lack of great teachers that talk in their own (real!) voices! One thing you should do, is talk with a sense of leadership. Really project your voice. It's also important to slow down (something I still struggle with). But keep your voice sounding like YOU! Authenticity is the backbone of any superhero.

Practice Karma Yoga

Another great way to get your practice hours (and confidence) up is to set up a free community 'karma yoga' class. Karma yoga is doing something without any expectation to receive anything in return. I never actually did this, but one of the teachers I mentored did, and I think it's really clever. She hired a church hall, made flyers, and ran free classes once a week. Her goal was to get used to leading a class in front of a group of strangers. The idea was a huge success.

Because the class is free it takes the pressure off you to be perfect, and sharing yoga from your heart in a room full of people is a wonderful way to experiment with your teaching sequences and style. Sadly, teaching for free may become unsustainable if teaching is going to be your main income, and very often people don't value what they get for free. However, karma yoga classes are a great 'baby step' towards charging for the real thing.

Collect Positive Feedback

Whenever I covered a class, if students approached me afterwards to thank me for the lesson or tell me they really enjoyed my class, I would always make a point of asking them if they can pass on any positive feedback to the manager and studio coordinator. (Remember, this is the person on whom you made a positive impact by taking the time to introduce yourself). As I will discuss later, the best form of advertising is word of mouth. It's important to be explicit because many people will rave about you to their friends but not to the people that can get you on the cover list. By making a point of specifically telling them how they can support you, it increases the chances massively of people actually following through.

As your confidence grows you will find that people will start asking you where else you teach. This is usually an indication that they really loved your class and would like it if you taught regular classes at a venue they can attend. Remember, don't be too timid here. Ask these students to tell the studio coordinator to give you a class if a slot appears. Then, as I mentioned earlier, always follow up with the studio coordinator. Write to them, or better still, find out who they are and go and tell him/her about some wonderful experiences you're having with the members. Be sincere about the positive feedback you've been receiving and tell them that a few students have asked if you will be given a regular slot.

Conversely, avoid being too pushy. How I often approached studio coordinators and centre managers when I first started teaching was to acknowledge that there must be lots of amazing teachers on the centre's waiting list, but that I'd love to be considered for any future classes that might come up. I can't stress enough the importance of HUMILITY! Humility doesn't mean thinking less of yourself, it just means you don't think you're more important than anyone else.

Cultivate Conscious Competence

If you start covering classes and feel like you're teaching bad classes, go easy on yourself. There is a stage in learning called 'conscious competence'. This is when you know what to do but you still have to think very consciously about every single step. With time and practice you will develop 'unconscious competence'. Where everything you say and do becomes second nature and you just flow effortlessly through the task.

The following example is what I often tell my students when they are learning challenging poses, and I think it is also appropriate here. If you were a parent and your baby was learning to walk, would you on its first few stumbles pull it to one side and tell him or her: *"Listen, I think this walking thing is not for you! Look, you tried a couple times and as you can see, you keep falling down. Maybe just stick to crawling, you're awesome at that."* Of course you wouldn't say that. You would give the child all the love, encouragement and guidance it needed. And what's more, you would give the baby endless opportunities to learn to walk.

Failure on the first few attempts is understandable because it's a new skill that you are developing. It doesn't mean that you are a failure! So if in the beginning you struggle to get classes or teach classes that aren't as good as Shiva Rae's, then keep going! Teach, teach, teach, teach, teach! The more you do this the better you'll get. With patience your super powers will emerge, but you have to believe in yourself. If you don't it'll show and it'll make it harder for others to believe in you too.

Private Clients

Private clients are an essential component to making ends meet as a yoga teacher. In some countries it is a rare concept, but here in the UK it is common that teachers build up a database of private clients. Getting private clients on your books is something that will start happening more regularly as you develop your skills as a teacher. I have found that students are usually keen to get a private teacher when they either don't have time to attend scheduled classes due to their hectic work schedule, or if they want to improve specific aspects of their practice in some way.

There are various things you can do to secure private clients…

Add Value

The most important thing you can do to acquire and retain private clients is to add value. When I first started teaching, I noticed that few teachers in London were breaking down more advanced postures into manageable steps to get the beginners progressing to an intermediate level, and the intermediate to advanced. I also realised that the teachers with the biggest followings would call out a couple of specific things to work on in each pose.

I quickly recognised that some students wanted specific pose 'breakdowns' and so began to teach in a manner that provided them with specific verbal cues and pose 'short cuts'. For example, in my first year of full-time teaching I was covering a class in a gym for a teacher whose style involved just calling each posture, but never verbalising tips on how to get the most out of the poses. Her style of teaching was immensely popular and the class was teaming with regular students. But there were some students in the class that were more beginner to intermediate level and making little mistakes that could be easily rectified if given additional verbal cues.

So although I was teaching a class that was similar to the regular teacher, with each posture I would give the students one simple thing to work on. For example, in Warrior 3, I told them to imagine someone was holding their leg and another onto their head, stretching them apart. Instantly everyone's Warrior 3 looked amazing. After the class finished several people came up to me and thanked me for a great class. They promised to tell the studio coordinator that they would love to have me as a regular teacher and I gained two private clients. Boom!

Have a Flexible Schedule

As you develop as a teacher and become more indemand, your students will fit into your schedule. In the beginning however, a great way to attract clients is to be available as much as possible. It is essential that you are willing to wake up earlier and go to bed later than anyone else to accommodate the schedules of your clients initially. Say goodbye to your weekends, evenings and all 'lieins' for the time being. Just like teaching classes, the more you teach privately the better you will become, and through word of mouth you will start gaining more students. Remember, being at your student's beck-and-call will not last forever. Trust that as your teaching super powers grow, so too will great opportunities. At some point you will be the master of your schedule and can limit your availability if you so choose.

Be Your Best Self

Always, no matter what, show up as your 'best self'. Be friendly and approachable (the two most important super powers). Be someone who is present when others are talking to you. Say nice things about other people when they aren't around, even if you don't agree with everything about them or the way they live their lives. Commend students on the effort they put it and make a point of specifically noting things that are impressing you about their progress. Finally, openly express your gratitude to everyone who attends your class. They are supporting you, when there are so many other incredible yoga superhero teachers out there. Remember that no matter how great you become, keep your feet on the ground and add value. By doing this you'll attract loyal private clients.

What to Charge

When I first started teaching I reached out to a few friends who were already established yoga teachers on the London scene to ask for advice about standard price points in the industry. One such teacher was my friend Beth. We sat down over a cup of tea one day and she asked me how my teaching was going. "It's actually going better than expected," I said with surprise. "I've even had some people ask me for private lessons!" She asked me what my next step was. "Well I thought I'd gain some experience teaching privates first, maybe teach for £30 for a few months and then slowly start to raise my fees as I impro…"

"That's way too cheap!" She cut me off. I tried to convince her otherwise but she was right and I knew it. A short while after we had this discussion I read a book I highly recommend, called "Influence" by Robert Caldini. In this book it explains that people equate how good something is with how much it costs. I realised that if I charged too little people would soon start thinking that I wasn't as good as other teachers who were charging more. Also, on a deep unconscious level, the more you charge the more value you will want to add into the client's lesson.

On a logistical level, you can only teach a certain amount of classes per day and per week. So you have to maximise how much you charge to help ease the amount of classes you need to make ends meet. I started my career with all guns blazing, running from client to client, teaching all day, every day. I quickly burnt out. Even worse was that I started losing clients and classes because I was simply too exhausted to give my best. I started taking short cuts in my teaching and I was foolish enough to think nobody would notice.

Beth also helped me to equate what I was doing with what other service driven jobs were charging per hour. "Let's look at massage for example." She explained. "Many massage therapists in spas charge in the range of £60 per hour and then the client is travelling to them. I always have to travel to my client's homes, so that adds hours of time lost on getting to and from the venue where no money can be earned." This simple point made me realise that it is extremely important to charge what you think you are worth. "If someone is not really willing to pay decent fees for private lessons, it's best to direct them to your group sessions until they can." Beth raised another valid point, "Once you have set the price, it's extremely hard to raise your fees later on," she wisely pointed out.

I know what you're thinking, "But this is such great chance to build my experience. How can I just refuse a paying client?" If you're pushed to accept an unacceptable offer, then go into the agreement making it clear that as you gain experience you will naturally begin to raise your fees. As yogi's we tend to be very giving and I've met many teachers who at times may attract people that take advantage of their generous spirit. Just because you teach yoga, it doesn't mean you have to give up all your possessions and become a monk. No, you are also entitled to a life of abundance.

Of course you can also go the other way, and I too made this mistake, by charging astronomical prices for one-hour sessions and in doing so lose some really loyal clients. Ask the teachers who you support what they charge to get an idea of the market rate. This will give you a gauge as to what is reasonable. Another good tip when someone is asking for your rates, is to name your price and then qualify that by asking, "Is that ok?" If it isn't you may want to meet the client half way and lower the cost, especially if you have the time and need more clients. As you become more and more busy you will not be able to afford the time for every client and class. You have to become selective. It is then that you have the freedom to decide which classes and clients are either the most fun, feasible or which are the best for your career progression.

As I became more established I found I had way too many clients. I simply couldn't afford the time to teach them all. So whenever any new clients asked for private lessons I would say, "I do take on new privates but at a much higher rate these days because I'm so busy." Then I would name the price. This immediately made it obvious that I was at a stage that saying "no" was more likely than me taking on another client at the same rate as my existing clientele. In this way I raised the level of my income slowly without maxing out my energy and teaching more. If anything, I cut back on classes and used the extra time to focus on developing the business aspect of my teaching.

Creating Mailing Lists

Collecting emails is one of the best ways to build your business. Once you have a student's email address you can start adding them to your mailing list (with permission and always with options to opt out if they choose). Consequently, after every class I invite interested students to share their email address with me so that they can receive my monthly newsletters. When I started teaching I couldn't ever imagine having enough to say to warrant creating a regular newsletter, so I wasn't diligent about saving the emails in one easy-to-find place and regret this in retrospect. Don't make my mistake!

Essentially, emails are the downward dog of marketing. As a tool it will give you the leverage to advertise your classes, workshops, retreats, events and more. Social media is another great marketing tool, but don't be fooled, email is king! Prioritise email over everything else. It is still the most effective form of marketing out there and if you build a following of loyal students, they will expect emails promoting your events.

One simple, but important point: if you're collecting emails in a notebook, always ask everyone to print their name legibly along with their email address, otherwise you run the risk of getting home and not being able to read messy writing. I usually give people my iPhone to type their name and email straight into my notebook app.

Call to Action

You've been using your yoga super powers for over an hour. The class has ended! Don't stop there! People want to be guided. This is your chance to give a 'call to action' to help elevate your career. I always announce any workshops, events or retreats I'm involved with at the end of class and specifically tell the students to come and ask me about the events. If I don't have any events coming up, I grow my email list by telling students to share their email address with me. Follow this up by making sure you give your students a clear call to action via email so they can sign up to upcoming happenings in advance. Offering incentives such as early bird rates is one great call to action method that encourages students to subscribe to your events with a sense of urgency.

Personalise

I really like personalising my newsletters by addressing each student by name. Many teachers write, 'Hey everyone!', or 'Hi my friends!', but I think it's more personal and effective to say, "Hi Sarah!" This can be tough if you have 500 names in your database, so explore using certain email database software programmes. I use Mail Chimp but do your own research to see which one you like. I like to think of all my students as individual little superhero's that I love and care about. Each one is special to me and I want them to feel that. So I make an effort to use people's names on email, in class and when I bump into them on the street.

Chapter 2

ELEVATE

Being in Flow

Ok my beautiful yoga superhero, your muscles are fired up and you've got your mojo flowing. Being midflow in your career means you're still working hard on your focus and growth but you are feeling unstoppable. Just like you picked up this book, I also felt like I needed a guide. Someone to show me what was possible. This is when help came from an unexpected place.

Vance was a receptionist at the first yoga centre I ever taught yoga at. He was taking a professional detour working at the centre but actually had a background in marketing and had a knack for customer service. We became friends and lucky for me, he took me under his wing after I told him I wanted to become a superhero. Over a few months he shared his extensive marketing insights and expertise with me, which inspired me to delve deeper into books on the topic and do more research online.

From that day onward, I kept learning and applying, learning and applying! I wanted to figure out what really works. And what doesn't. In addition to helping my career, I shared what I knew with other yoga teachers and started seeing transformation happening in the teachers around me. This practical, handson approach was the key to my marketing success and helped elevate me, and my yoga career, to the next level.

In this chapter I want to 'pay-it-forward' by sharing what I did with the help from Vance, the resources I read and the things I put into practice.

Teaching in Yoga Centres

When I first started teaching yoga I broke into the industry by spreading my time between a few gyms and a community centre. But my goal was to get into a dedicated yoga centre. The only problem was I had no idea how to get myself on the timetable when there were so many other yoga teachers in London with more experience than I had.

Many new teachers face this dilemma and depending what your goals are, you might be happy to stick to your gym classes. My personal goal was to reach a wider audience. Being in a respected yoga studio not only gave me more access to students who specifically want to advance in yoga; but it also put me 'on the map'. Perception is everything when it comes to marketing yourself to students. The teachers in yoga centres are not necessarily better than the teachers in gyms, but there is a certain reputation that comes with saying you teach in a top yoga centre. I was aware of this fact to a certain degree but when it really became clear to me was when I was teaching my second retreat. I was casually chatting to all the attendees at the dinner table when one student asked me where I taught (you get asked this question more than any other). When I told her, she immediately commented on how that is how she knows whether a teacher is good or not. I asked her what she meant and she said, *"because it's so difficult to get into top yoga centres, if you're a teacher there you must be good"*. All this was from a woman who had done only a handful of yoga classes in her whole life.

Manage Your Media Image

So how do you make the transition from amateur to superhero? The first step is to get a kickass website up and running which showcases the very best of you. Social media also helps and later in the book I'll outline ways to gain a healthy number of followers. The book, *'Influence'* I mentioned earlier addresses a very interesting concept called 'social proof'. According to the law of social proof, if you see lots of people doing something you will automatically think it is a good thing to do.

For example, have you ever been on holiday looking for a good place to eat and favoured a certain place because it was full of people? I know I have. Who's to say whether that restaurant is better or not? The truth is you don't really know. What you do know is that you are using social proof to make these conclusions. As you gain more followers on social media, people will equate how good you are with how popular you are.

I know, you might be thinking that we live in a sad, superficial world if that is how we rate and equate quality. And while I tend to agree on some level, I also believe social media is an invaluable marketing tool and is where the future of marketing lies.

If you want to do social media, then do it well! You'll be amazed at the difference it will make to your career.

Trade Shows

Once you have a great website and healthy social media following, start applying to teach at every trade show under the sun. First of all, to gain experience, but also so that ultimately you can teach at yoga trade shows or other yoga festivals in the future. I remember being desperate to raise my game and move away from gyms and into yoga centres. So the very first opportunity I had to teach at the Yoga Show in the UK, I grabbed it. Before my class I went to the yoga centres that had stands and connected with the people who worked there. I asked them if they would like to come along to my class to see me teach as it was my dream to be on their cover list.

The key aspect of this tactic is that I made it clear I wanted to be on their *cover list* (not their regular list). This shows you're realistic and willing to work hard. I had no expectation that they would actually attend my class, but they actually did come along and the following Monday I had an email in my inbox offering me a place on their cover list. I was over the moon!

This kind of initiative never goes unnoticed. Even if for some reason they don't follow through, trust me, you've made a lasting impression on them.

The yoga world is actually very small, so if you bump into them again, chances are they'll remember you.

Social Networking

Another way to get into yoga centres is to get to know as many people as possible. You'll soon start to realise that everyone knows everyone in the yoga community, and that interconnectedness will work for or against you one day. When I was getting started on my journey into yoga centres I was asked, along with a bunch of other teachers, to help a superhero yoga teacher in London with one of her events. I jumped at the chance with no thought of what was in it for me and I really gave it my all.

However I was amazed at the attitude of the other teachers. Many complained constantly, didn't show up, asked for compensation for their time and didn't give their best. The reason I was shocked at their attitudes was that it was their choice to join in the event. Nobody forced them into it. My philosophy was, and still is, that once I commit I have to give 100%, even if I wasn't going to get anything in return. So I made sure I was on time and professional. I never complained and did my best with everything, including offering to help in any additional way that I could.

It paid off too. Once the event had passed and the dust had settled, the teacher running the event, sent an apology email to all the teachers for not providing enough compensation for their time, and asked if there was some way she could repay them. I jumped at the chance. I wrote to her sincerely praising her efforts and all the success of the event and told her that if I could, I would do it all again. I was genuinely grateful for having had the opportunity to get involved with her event. In addition to expressing my gratitude I asked her if she would mind connecting me to one of the yoga centres where she teaches.

I explained that breaking into these environments is a huge challenge for a new teacher and was one of my goals. Within the hour she connected me to the studio manager and a trial was arranged.

Connect to the Wider Community

Growing as a teacher doesn't mean you have to be an island. It involves connecting with the wider yoga community and using established superhero's as a platform to give you a helping hand. By being present, helping and supporting others and doing it with a smile you will put the law of reciprocation into place. This law states that if you do something for someone else, even if it's just a small gesture, the chances are that person will feel obliged on some level to reciprocate.

I personally don't go around helping people with the mentality that they should help me back. In my mind I've altered this law slightly. I believe that if you help someone else you will have something great come your way. Maybe not from that person, maybe from a totally unexpected person, place or thing, but generally what you give is what you get.

Name Dropping

Another great idea is to start 'name dropping'. Not you specifically, but your students and loyal fans. Whenever I had a student come up to me and express their appreciation for my classes I would ask them to please tell the yoga centres that they attend about me, either through comment cards or an email. I did this a few times in various centres and it wasn't long before I had the yoga managers attending my classes to see what I was all about. I never wasted my time sending a cover letter and a CV. The best way to connect to top studios, in my opinion, was to get other people singing my praises.

Connecting to Brands

Another invaluable piece of advice Vance gave me was to connect to established brands that are active in the yoga community. It is important to create contact with brands whose philosophies resonate with you and that you are passionate about. The key is just that: be passionate about the brand and show keen and sincere excitement. Be present at all their events and community classes. Connect with them via social media and get to know and support the team members that work for your chosen brand. The incredible individuals that work for various companies in the industry are always on the lookout for local yoga superhero's that can elevate their brand.

How do you achieve this? Send 100 emails if you have

to. Find out what the values of the company are and think of creative ways to support them. Go and meet people face-to-face. I became a brand ambassador for lululemon because I spent time with, and befriended the people who ran the brand's showrooms. They were all really lovely people who had a passion for helping others. I also created a relationship with the yoga mat company Liforme. The founder graciously contacted me, and soon after an organic friendship formed.

Link to people through brands and you'll be amazed at what opportunities come your way. Connecting to brands is an effective way to grow as a teacher in your community. Make an effort to find brands whose ethos speak to you. Even if what you expected doesn't happen, perhaps you make new friends, introduce other people and fellow teachers and help them grow, or you could get cool tips on how to make your own brand stand out.

Action Point:
Now it's time for you to do something!

Research three brands whose ethos you love and write to them. Find out how you can support them and get to know some of the people working for the company. Figure out the company goals and see if any align with yours. See if you can connect with them and get a face-to-face meeting with a brand representative.

This exercise is in here not so that you can go and impress

people or even get something from them, it's about learning to reach out beyond your comfort zone. Even if connecting with these brands doesn't yield anything, you will end up meeting some key people in your field that can inspire you.

I remember attending one of the community classes for lululemon and the owner of a top London yoga centre was teaching. I approached her after class, expressing how much I enjoyed the session and told her that it was my goal to start teaching in yoga centres. She said that the only way teachers are recruited into her centre was if they completed the teacher training that they ran. I promised that I would research it and do my utmost to attend. Although at the time I couldn't afford the fee, so I left it there.

Months later I saw the same lady again at an event and I asked her how her business was going. I also expressed my sincere admiration for her ability to simultaneously teach and run a studio. She opened up and started sharing some of the challenges she was facing, telling me how difficult it was to do both and how challenging it was to find good cover teachers. I offered to connect her to some of the wonderful teachers I use for cover, which she accepted.

A few months later I bumped into her and her business partner and they expressed just how great the suggested teachers had been. On the spot the two of them invited me to run a workshop in their centre in London and another one in their Birmingham centre. They even offered me classes in their centre. Despite not having done a single course run through them I managed to gain workshops and teaching opportunities. The lesson? Be persistent! Don't give up at the first hurdle if the brands or opportunities that you seek out aren't responsive. Keep at it and always put your best foot forward. You never know what could come about from just one new relationship.

Creating a Brand

Creating my own brand was something I did very early on in my career. I wanted to create something that was not linked to my name, but a separate stand-alone brand that didn't need my face to run it. I was criticised for this, as all the big names in the yoga industry were using their personal names as their branding and marketing tools. But in my mind I saw it as an opportunity to create a little business. This is what a real business does: it creates an income when you're not there. If your business is only generating a salary if you are present, then you don't own a business, you own a job. This was also based on advice that was passed down to me from various business mentors which led me to believe that using another name was pivotal for the longevity of a business. However, now that I am living off the royalties produced by my name I realise that perhaps there are exceptions to the rule.

My first brand was called "Yoga Heaven". I chuckle to myself admitting this to you. I spent about three days on Google searching for various company names and it is amazing how everything with the name yoga seems to have been taken. Then after a lot of frustration I keyed in Yoga Heaven and the URL was available (probably because most people thought it was terrible name). Because my name "Celest", means heaven, in my mind this name made perfect sense. So off I trotted and made a logo and got business cards printed. I thought this was a brilliant name, but very quickly received feedback from various people telling me my branding wasn't targeted enough and didn't have legs. I took a long, hard look at my brand name to decide if their advice was something that would serve me or not. In hindsight I think people didn't have the heart to tell me that Yoga Heaven was a tacky name and that it sucked! In the end I realised that Yoga Heaven was not for me and I began the search for something stronger.

Around about that time I started reading the book, *'Key Person of Influence'* by Daniel Priestly. This book advises you to find a 'micro-niche' within a niche. In the yoga realm, yoga is the niche and a micro-niche is a specialty such as prenatal yoga, yoga for teenagers, or acroyoga. Either way, find a group within a group to cater to. Whenever I mentor teachers on finding their micro-niche I sense there is a lot of fear in making this decision. Mainly because they don't want to pigeon hole themselves or their services. I normally ask them, "Who is your target audience?" And the common answer I receive is "Everyone!" While I understand why people want to cater to a wide spectrum of people and are afraid of excluding anyone or limiting their potential clients, being too generic can work to your disadvantage when it comes to marketing your brand. Because although everyone can benefit from yoga, you can't *market* to everyone. Different people have different needs and require different messages.

After much deliberation I rebranded to 'cityogi'. My main reason for this was because I decided my microniche was to teach urban professionals. A concept that made complete sense in London where there is a massive group of people who work in the city and are seeking recreational activities to help them cope with the stresses of city life. I found my fire burned the brightest when I was teaching this demographic. They were motivated in class, so I could take them to an advanced level of practice in a short space of time. They also loved seeing the measurable results, but all of them reported being more present and peaceful post class, and this made me feel like I was making a difference.

By specialising in a specific niche you can position yourself as the 'go-to' person for that particular specialty. A common mistake many new teachers make is that they become addicted to adding new feathers to their yoga bow, instead of concentrating on one type or form. As the old saying goes 'Jack of all Trades, Master of None'; this is true for many new teachers who are qualified to teach everything from vinyasa flow to Iyengar and restorative, yet lack a specific forte.

While it's great to do courses and have extra knowledge, if you position yourself in the community as a teacher that can teach anything to anyone you'll never get known for a particular skill set. In a sea of teachers there you are, just one of countless waves bobbing up and down. I'm not saying you should exclude anyone from your classes who doesn't fit your ideal customer profile, but you should put time and energy into creating a brand that makes you stand out from the crowd. To do that you need to be known for a type of yoga and in the back of your mind cater to a specific type of person.

Defining a Customer Profile

After you have chosen the type of yoga you love teaching, have a think about what type of people you would love to work with. Are they male or female? Where do they work? Where do they live? What do your ideal customers like to do? Are they married? Do they have kids? Where do they shop? What other forms of activity do they like other than yoga? Remember, this is an 'ideal world' scenario. Who are your dream clients? Remember, just because you have ideal clients and a chosen form of practice that you wish to be known for, doesn't mean you'll be restricting yourself. It'll just give you direction. If you choose to incorporate other styles into your class to spice things up, go for it! And if people who don't fit your ideal customer base turn up, you don't have to send them away. This exercise just helps you define your branding and makes you more targeted in your business approach.

Exercise

Take some time now to write an ideal customer profile. Name them, give them an address and describe them in detail. I spent a good hour on this when I first started out, and wrote pages and pages of information. It made making decisions about logos, website colours, products and style much easier.

Creating a Logo

Once you have completed creating a picture of who your customer is, you can mould your branding to compliment that demographic.

Choosing a logo is a great starting point. E-lance (www.elance.com) and 99Designs (www.99designs.com) are two super cool companies that you can use to design a logo. These companies have loads of designers on their database that compete for your money. For example, with 99Designs, when you decide to host a 'contest', you pay a fee (which is refundable if you don't get back a design that you like) while the designers compete to impress you with their designs. As they compete you can give them feedback and tell them what you like and what you don't. As your feedback comes in they continually update the designs until you find the design that you like best.

When I started Yoga Heaven I asked my friend, who is an artist, to create my first logo and it was really great. Afterwards I used 99Designs (where you can get many styles of designers working for you), but I've heard E-lance are just as good. The next step is creating a website. I'll talk more about that later on in the chapter, but for now know that a good website is a huge help in taking you to the next level.

Embracing Change

Once my Cityogi brand was up and running, I realised that although I loved teaching city professionals, what was really lighting my fire, was that I could teach them the advanced aspects of yoga whilst adding in my own spin on self-development and spirituality. It was then that I expanded my vision. I started using my own name in branding myself as a teacher, and my demographic shifted to a more modern yoga audience – people who love yoga movement and the lifestyle, with a unique fresh, curious view of the philosophy. I also expanded into catering products for yoga teachers that were getting started on their careers, hence the creation of this book.

This demographic, in my eyes, needed help in learning how to break into the yoga industry and also how to approach some of the more advanced yoga poses. The beauty of having your own brand and business is that you can change your mind! So if you start out teaching pregnant women but suddenly feel your calling is actually acroyoga, you can change. Never feel like your brand is a fixed entity. It's as flexible as you want it to be. At the same time be careful not to abandon ship at any given whim. You need to keep your mind focused on the goal and find a way of getting your brand to work you toward that.

Creating Online Content

In recent years, writing articles, blog posts, filming content and shooting images has become an important marketing tool for the modern yogi. In the same way that a good brand name, website and logo help build a brand image, creating yoga-related content is a great way to cultivate an online connection with your clients (and potential clients!), and to share your 'voice' in the yoga community. In relation to writing, I would simply shut down. My dyslexia presented huge challenges for me so the thought of writing an article that could be read and critiqued in a public forum was truly terrifying. And yet, here I am, a published writer, writing a book. Believe me, if I can do it, you can do it!

One of the main mental obstacles I had when I thought about creating content was not knowing what to create. I didn't think I knew anything of significant value that other people would want to know, or could learn from. But that's simply not true. Each and every one of us has unique thoughts, opinions, insights, perspectives and experiences, which are worthy of sharing with others. Nobody on this planet has had your life experience or your perspective. Every struggle, mistake and heartache was there to teach you something. What you know now could give someone else hope that they are not alone in what they are facing.

So create something! Even if it's short and sweet and to the point. What has inspired you recently? How has it made you change the way you think or act? What is the best piece of advice you were ever given? How have you made a difference in other people's lives and how did that effect you?

To overcome my initial deer-in-headlights writing paralysis, I decided to write about a topic that was close to my heart: happiness. More specifically, I asked myself the question, *"What is it that makes me a happy person?"* The answers came quickly and effortlessly and I started writing them down. Before long, my personal happiness-inducing list had tuned into my first article. And the best part is, I enjoyed writing it! I posted the article on my website, after which a website called 'All My Goodness' (www.allmygoodness.com) re-posted it, followed by American website 'Yoga Download' (www.yogadownload.com), after which respected UK publication 'Om Yoga & Lifestyle Magazine' (www.ommagazine.com) published it. All of these platforms indirectly gave me free advertising simply because I wrote about what I'm good at: being happy!

The more you create content of various forms and put it up, the more Google will love you and bump you up the rankings. Write from your heart and regularly send your best work to magazines and blogging sites. Or create videos or audio programmes (more on that later). Once you have something published with your name, website and article appearing in more than one place on the web, Google will automatically rank your URL higher. There's no question that improving your writing skills, videography and photography skills is an essential part of building your name.

The key to writing is not to write in a fancy way that makes the reader wish he or she had a dictionary close by, but to write in a conversational tone, as if you are giving a good friend advice. There's no point being profound if no-one can relate to you! Instead, be real. People appreciate and connect to raw honesty.

Similarly if you are filming content, talk in your authentic voice. Be yourself! Be honest about your challenges and strengths, and imagine you're chatting to a friend. The more natural you are, the more people will respond positively to the content you create.

The second key to launching and running a successful blog/vlog (video log) is consistency. Posting a regular blog entry on your website is key to good Search Engine Optimisation (SEO is how well your website ranks in search engines), and feeds your followers with fresh content. Google loves it when you have new content popping up all the time and your followers (potential clients!) will be more likely to subscribe to your site or blog if you post interesting material regularly. Ideally, you should be posting content at least once a week, preferably on the same day, so as your followers know when to expect new content.

Going Viral

Another effective way of getting your blog exposed is to write a blog post in 'reply' format to a post that is trending. If you read the big journal articles that are getting attention and have a strong opinion on the topic, then write about it. Take note of where that person's blog is being featured, tweeted and posted, then post your website's URL with a comment on the topic. This will do wonders for your website's SEO.

Also, don't be afraid to be controversial! I created a YouTube video once describing why doing hero pose is bad for your knees. Even now as you read this a strong opinion one way or the other will pop into your mind. Well that video got lots of attention! Both positive and negative. Many people shared the video and commented on the fact that what I was saying made sense. While others posted about me in teaching forums saying I was stupid and didn't know what I was talking about. Either way, I got lots of traffic to my site and lots of work came my way off the back of being a little controversial.

Getting online exposure really helps raise your profile as a teacher. This is useful, not because more people will think how great you are, but simply because more people will hear your message. Remember that your message is powerful and has the ability to make someone else's life better. Doing things beyond your comfort zone helps you exceed your own expectations of what you thought you were capable of.

Your Message

One of the most important questions you need to ask yourself before embarking on your teaching journey is: *What is your message?* What is it that you want to share with people in your classes, articles and social media posts? Do you want to pass down ageold yoga philosophies, or do you have unique modern insights that you feel can add value to people's lives? It is really important to make your mind up about what it is that you want to share with the world, then commit to sharing this openly and freely. Never underestimate your message. It is valuable beyond measure.

Choose Your Medium

Choosing a medium that works for you and your personality is vital to online success. If you're a writer, write blog posts and tweets. If you're great on camera, film YouTube videos or host an online webinar. If you're a photographer, get on Instagram. Choose a medium through which you can deliver great quality and add value. Whatever you choose, become great at it. Take note of what gets high interaction with your followers. Are the articles with lots of shares touching on controversial topics? Or is it your quirky sense of humour that's resonating with people? Once you recognise what works then make it your own and stick to what is aligned to your values.

Experimentation is the key. I am still relatively small on social media, but even with my tiny reach, I've had a multitude of work come my way, simply because I have some level of presence on social media. I also now stick to mediums that I enjoy working on. There are only so many hours in the day, so spending time on every medium under the sun is counter productive. I now focus my time on video and photography because I am super passionate about creating great, engaging content with these two mediums.

Teaching Workshops

Teaching workshops is a great way to connect to your students in a deeper way. The added bonus is that workshops are little cash injection that takes the pressure off making ends meet. You might be thinking that talking about money as a yoga teacher is not being spiritual. That may be true, but remember, often balancing the books as a yoga teacher can be challenge, and this stress can have a negative effect on your health and career. If you want to keep teaching, then use your passion to live a kick ass, free from money stress life.

That said, don't just teach workshops to make a quick buck. It's important to see workshops as a chance to give people an opportunity to learn something new that they won't get the chance to learn in a normal shortform class setting. For the longest time I thought I had nothing to offer that was unique compared to other teachers. This is simply not true. Your perspective is uniquely yours, and therefore it is your job to become aware of the value of your unique perspective and to learn how to express it to your students. The most important thing by far is to BE YOURSELF!

When I began teaching workshops I remember feeling insecure about the content I was sharing. Consequently, I felt obligated to add many traditional aspects of yoga into my workshops, including chanting, mudras, breathing and postures. I put in everything and the kitchen sink. But as my confidence grew I realised that I wasn't being fully authentic (to myself!). What I loved more about yoga was the movement, anatomy and self-development aspects of the practice. When I started becoming more honest with myself about what I really loved and what was making a positive impact on my life, my workshops started getting busier. What's more, studios from all over London and neighbouring cities started inviting me to teach for them.

Finding Your Signature Style

Finding a signature style that distinguishes your teaching technique from the many other teachers out there is an important part of refining your niche. Identifying what makes you and your teaching different to other people's is an extremely important aspect of brand-building too. So step outside your comfort zone! Stop teaching like your teacher taught you and be original.

For me personally, I love the challenge of difficult postures and used my own practice to explore interesting ways to break poses down into 'baby steps' so that I could become stronger or more flexible. There weren't many teachers who were taking the time to do this in their classes when I started out, so I decided to bring this step-by-step posture break down to my classroom. Some people loved this new approach and others hated it. Many people wanted to be led through a class full of postures they could already do without pushing themselves too hard; while others loved seeing their physical practice progress. The latter group would shout my name loudly in class while balancing precariously in an upside down position, to make sure that I didn't miss the first time they did a pose they never thought they would ever do. Yet in some studios this style of teaching was making me lose students fast. This led me to question my abilities as a teacher, and for a while I conformed and returned to the 'safer' teaching style, without the posture breakdowns. But it wasn't long before I felt deeply unfulfilled and without even consciously thinking about it, I was breaking postures down again.

When I made the transition from gyms into yoga centres this skill was refined and finally I was in the right environment to flourish. I was given the opportunity to teach in a style that suited me and got a great response from students. Students started to progress and class numbers grew. And of course, this skill was what people came to my workshops for. It became my signature style. Students knew that a bit more time with me meant they could walk out doing something they couldn't do when they walked in. Teaching in an authentic style made me feel like the superhero of my world. Nothing will empower you more than doing what you love and being yourself each and every day.

How to Structure a Workshop

When you first start teaching workshops, one of the most daunting thoughts is *"How am I going to fill all that time?!"* I was petrified of this and frequently had nightmares about getting to the end of my content with a full hour left. The way to get around this is to attend other workshops and scribble ideas down. Everything from how the teacher structured the workshop to what they spent more time on and how they involved the students.

Something that helped me was to break my workshops down into sections. I chose what I know and love: yoga, advanced postures, self-development, and meditation. Then I would choose a theme that suited all of these. For example, if I was teaching arm balances, I would speak about the 'circle of comfort' and I would show that yoga had the ability to expand this circle in every direction. I would then tell a story related to confidence and then I would add these concepts into the meditation at the end.

Armed with all of this, I taught my heart out. With whatever time was left, I would have a few different ideas in my back pocket that I could bring out in case I still had any spare time left over. For example, I would include specific stretches related to the topic and alignment tips from my physiotherapy background. Planning is the key, and then like everything, just doing it! You may not be great at it in the beginning, but who cares? You're putting yourself out there and learning a great deal in the process.

Workshop Do's and Don'ts

If you are going to teach a workshop, take the time to prepare properly. Remember people have spent their precious time and money on a workshop with you, so be professional and show up ready to add great value. Please don't be one of those yoga teachers who stretches out a yoga class to make it longer and have the nerve to call it a workshop. I once went to a workshop led by a popular international teacher and all he did was practice on his mat, calling the poses from start to finish. He didn't add any value to the class and I left wanting more. On the flip side, when Irene Pappas (www.fitqueenirene.com) came to London, she took the time to go from person to person asking if there was anything they wanted to learn that day.

And Chris Chavez (www.chrischavez.com), gave me the awesome idea of getting all the students to put large name labels on their mats so he could call them by their names. Dylan Werner was a master at bringing something unique and special to the workshops and was constantly present with the people in the room. Always take the time to notice how the students are responding to what you are teaching, and then take the time to modify what you are doing to suit the room. Break students off into groups to talk through concepts or practice postures. Acknowledge how well students are doing along the way to keep them inspired and get students of all skill levels to demonstrate for the group. I love choosing beginners to demonstrate. It really breaks the definition of what a 'skilled yogi' looks like.

I once listened to a TED talk about leadership, where the speaker said that if you can highlight the positive aspects of what students are doing well you'll raise the level of all the students in the room because they will begin to understand what it is that will propel them forwards. As opposed to avoiding the things that you noted as being wrong.

Getting people to attend your workshop can be another challenge. As I grew as a teacher, I started getting many offers to teach workshops in various places. I loved teaching them but what I found really exhausting was the marketing. There's no doubt about it... the amount of time you spend planning and marketing workshops is immense, and can sometimes take as much time and energy as the workshop itself.

Teaching Retreats

Teaching retreats are another fun, exciting way to earn money as a teacher and share a deeper side of what you have to offer. Because you are with the same group for an extended period of time, you have the opportunity to see your students grow day after day.

Retreat Preparation

Good preparation is the key to running a successful retreat. Having an outline of how you would like to see the group progress is an important first step when it comes to structuring a timetable. And yet, you also need to be prepared to throw your planned itinerary out the window, as you never know what the group dynamic is going to be or what challenges are going to present themselves. Be mindful of what you enjoy teaching and be prepared to come up with creative ways of getting the group to discover these things.

Make sure that the first day is a gentle ease into the retreat. Yoga twice a day is very intense and if students get really sore on the first day, they might be more susceptible to injury as the week goes on. Gradually build up the sessions. Also have spare fun ideas ready. I once taught a group that found my style of teaching way too challenging for their level. So I got them to do lots of partner work, a great way to keep up morale and get them learning. I also did an alignment workshop, a goal-setting workshop and a beach class. Combining all these ideas meant that I could create a memorable experience for the attendees whist staying true to what I loved to teach.

Bond With Your Students

When you're on your retreat, be present. What do I mean? Some yoga teachers only turn up for the classes they have to teach, then disappear the rest of the time. It is important to take time away from the group to recharge your energy, but you can also gain energy by hanging out with your students and getting to know them. If you disagree with this statement, I accept that. But remember this retreat is not a holiday, it's work. So don't get complacent. The students are all special people that have chosen you and your style of teaching to help them progress in their practice and their lives. This is a greatest compliment and it is important that you value and cherish the time (and money!) they have taken to spend with you on the retreat. If you take the time to hang out with the participants on your retreat you will find the same people will come back year after year after year. This is how you grow a loyal following and a sustainable business.

My current retreats are not just filled with loyal students, but with great friends, who I bonded with on past retreats. I feel so proud that some of the students that have met on my retreats are now best friends and we often hang out on the weekend or go out to dinner together. In my personal opinion the biggest superhero's are the people that really take time to connect to other people and make their students feel like superhero's too.

Retreat Logistics

The best way to get advice about the best places to lead retreats and learn about retreat do's and don'ts is to talk to other yoga teachers in your community. Ask them about what worked, what didn't, and why. Ask them about their favourite locations and whether they'd mind connecting you to these places. This is the easiest way to find venues that host retreats.

Be aware that running retreats yourself can be intense because you are acting as the teacher and travel agent. Be prepared to answer lots of mundane questions and deal with everything from people's dietary requests to their sleeping arrangements. Subsequently, it is important you price the retreat so you are earning two salaries for the week, not just one. Many teachers undersell themselves. Remember, people equate the amount they're paying to the value you'll deliver. So don't feel bad to charge what you feel you are worth. Just make sure you deliver value beyond what you charge them, and they'll walk away raving. Personally, I love running retreats myself, but I do find them much more time-intensive.

If you don't want the hassle of handling finances, bookings, flights and transfers, you can run your retreat through a yoga retreat agency. There are plenty of specialised companies who run yoga holidays all over the globe. This is a really easy way to run retreats as they often help you market your retreat and handle bookings, so you don't have to do it all by yourself. However it's important to make sure the agency profit-share structure is a win/win for all involved, otherwise your profits will end up in someone else's pocket.

Theming Your Retreat

When I first started running retreats I was worried that nobody would book or turn up, so I said yes to everyone who wanted to come along. But that made it more difficult to help everyone progress at their level. I had some super advanced people and some total beginners. A great way to avoid this issue is to theme the retreat to give people an idea of what to expect. The theme should be broad enough so nobody feels excluded, yet specific enough to appeal to a niche clientele. For example, my favourite theme is 'Advance Your Practice'. This gives my audience the impression that no matter what level they are, they will be doing a physical practice that will involve lots of postures they might not yet be able to do yet. The theme shows potential attendees that we will have a strong physical practice to look forward to.

Marketing Yourself

You can be the best yoga teacher on the planet, but if people don't know about you or where you are teaching, then your super heroness might only reach a very small group of people. Marketing is not my passion. Teaching is my passion. But if I'm teaching to an empty room then I can't follow my passion, so over the years I've made a concerted effort to educate myself about effective marketing tools. There are so many different types of marketing out there which can be really overwhelming if you don't have a background in marketing (which I don't) and aren't used to promoting yourself. When I started out I knew nothing about marketing and made a lot of mistakes. And you know what, I still do! But being out there, mistakes and all, has attracted a great little tribe of people who I love.

Although promoting yourself might feel a tad 'unyogic', it's a necessary part of survival as a teacher. In my heart I want to help people through my teaching. I want lots of people to hear my message, so I do my utmost to reach the biggest audience possible and don't feel bad about learning and applying marketing strategies so that more people can find out about me and my teachings. I also see this time we are living in right now as a great privilege. We can market ourselves with little or no budget. A few years ago this was impossible. Remember this quote, "you can either hate the game, or play the game!" or like my good friend Marc said, "or you can create the game."

Eight Simple Steps to Good Marketing

Since I knew nothing about marketing when I first launched my brand, I took an online marketing course with a great coach named Brendon Burchard (www.brendonburchard.com), who distilled effective marketing down to eight simple steps. These easy-to-follow guidelines help draw people to your message and have made a huge (positive!) difference to my personal branding strategy.

1. **Claim** - What will your class, retreat or workshop do for the attendees. By gaining the knowledge that you have to share, how will this knowledge impact their lives?

2. **Challenges** - What are the common challenges that they may face along the way?

3. **Commonality** - How are you like your students? What did you have to overcome to get to where you are now?

4. **Credibility** - What have you achieved that qualifies you to teach this particular thing.

5. **Choice** - What other classes are out there and how does yours compare? Why is your course the intelligent course?

6. **Comparison Pricing** - What would it cost the students elsewhere? Why is the course with you such a deal?

7. **Concerns** - What concerns do your clients have? Money? Time? Injuries? Families?

8. **Call to action** - Always direct them to where you want them to go next. If it's at the end of class ask for their email. If it's to buy a ticket to your workshop on an email, say CLICK HERE!

Social Media

Social media might not be your passion, however it is an excellent way of raising your profile for free. It does take a lot of time and hard work, and initially might feel like you're stabbing away in the dark, but once you find the right medium and begin to see your social media following grow that will inspire you to continue and keep it going.

Three years after I started teaching full time I decided to read a book about social media to learn how to grow my network. Really this should have been one of the very first things that I did when I started my career. It would have halved the time it took me to get access to teaching in big events like the Yoga Show, or in quality yoga centres. I know it feels fickle and like a big popularity contest. But I like to think of life as a fun game with rules (that can be broken), 'get of jail' cards, bonus rounds and surprises with each roll of the dice. I don't take anything too seriously. Mostly because my yoga journey has taught me that nothing is really real. It's all an illusion, or in my case a game. As I said earlier, you can play the game and have some fun, or fight against it and cause yourself stress. I like to have fun!

Building a Following on Social Media

There is no social media magic wand. Building a social media following takes a great deal of time, effort and dedication. To see your social media strategy work, YOU have to work, however the key to growing a strong social media following was summed up to me by my two friends Alex and Mimi Ikonn (both social media superhero's) in four simple letters: QVCA. Let me elaborate…

Quality

Whatever you create should be high quality. I mentioned this earlier in the book, whatever medium you choose to focus on, make it great. For example, I chose YouTube and Instagram as mediums to grow my online presence. So I began to research how to take great pictures and make fun videos for my profile. I also invested in a good camera to film my YouTube videos and later a microphone and some lights (which can be bought cheaply on Ebay) to make sure my sound and picture quality was good. You don't need lots of fancy tricks, backgrounds, or even different camera angles. But a good image with lots of light and good sound should be the aim for anyone running a YouTube channel.

Value

V stands for value. In life, the more value you give freely, the more opportunities will come your way. Earlier in the book I explained the concept of 'process of reciprocation'. Where, if you do something for someone else, or give them something for no reason, there is a strong possibility they will want to reciprocate. Well, when you add value on social media, you start to tap into this law on a much larger scale. Don't think about how rich this is going to make you, just focus on how much value you are adding to others.

Consistency

This is where most people fall short. To do well on any social media network, you have to release consistent content. This consistency is what brings back old followers and creates new ones. But of course, anything with a regular release schedule can be difficult to maintain. When I first launched my YouTube channel, I released only one or two videos and thought that would help accentuate my superhero status. Around that time I met Alex and Mimi who kindly told me, "you're doing it all wrong!". I then started releasing one new video each and every week. There were many weeks when this was tough, because making a simple YouTube video takes hours, but the effort translated into followers and eventually it attracted other opportunities.

Authenticity

Authenticity is the most important part of any endeavour (you'll hear me say this again and again). This is especially true when it comes to your social media persona. People can usually spot a fake a mile away so don't be afraid to be your self. The little quirky mistakes that you make are what people will love. Your human 'flaws' will help people relate to you. When I first started teaching, I was waaaaaay too formal in my approach. My desire to be 'yogic', calm and serene was preventing my true self from shining which was holding my YouTube channel back. So I started to relax and let my bubbly personality come out to play more. The effect was immediate, not only did I feel more 'myself', but my subscriber list doubled in a few months.

Also, be prepared to share your struggles in life. I personally found that being open and honest about what I can't do, the mistakes I've made and the challenges I am faced with, help people to get to know me. Remember, people would rather support people they know. So allow people to get to know that becoming a superhero takes time, by sharing your story.

Other Social Media Do's & Don'ts
Separate Your Platforms

Many teachers link up all of their social media platforms to minimise the time they spend advertising the same thing. Although I can see the benefits of this, books on social media warn against it and encourage people to battle all platforms as separate beasts. The main reason for participating in social media is to ENGAGE your audience. All platforms have their own little rules to follow. So if you've linked up Instagram and Twitter your tweet will not appear in full and the image will appear as a link.

Ultimately you want your social media to be 'sticky'. You want people to visit it again and again and feel compelled to interact with your content. This might make it less appealing to your audience. Also avoid sharing the same content on all.

Don't Over-Promote

Don't use social media to self-promote all the time. If your only content is a promotion about your next workshop or a review about how wonderful your latest retreat was, you're going to lose followers fast. Instead, enrich people with interesting information about what is going on in the wider yoga community. Ask provocative questions that will stir conversation and stimulate interaction between your followers. Connect your audience to resources that are inspiring you.

A good tip that I picked up from reading the book, *'The Impact Equation'*, by Chris Brogan and Juliet Stanwell Smith, is to think of all social media platforms as a party. You wouldn't walk up to a stranger at a party and give them a stack of your business cards asking him or her to hand them out to their friends. The idea is ridiculous right? So don't bother doing it on social media either.

Instagram

Taking beautiful shots and videos and sharing inspirational sentiments around what that image represents on Instagram is something that my personal audience has responded well to. In my classes I encourage people to feel good about their bodies, and about who they are and what they can do. That is why I take images of yoga postures that will inspire people to get onto the mat and love themselves fully. I also do my best to add lots of value by sharing what I do daily to be healthy and happy.

I made the mistake, early on, of using too many hash tags on my posts. It's best to avoid this for a few reasons, the main one being, because it distracts from the key message of the post and can make your post look like messy spam. However, if used the right way hashtags can also help you grow your following, but only if they are actually seen, so avoid adding a generic tag such as #Yoga, or your post will be lost in a matter of seconds. One way you can leverage hashtags is to create a few key hashtags and save them in your notes folder on your phone. Instead of placing them on your actual post put them in a comment straight underneath your post. That way as you gain more comments the hashtags disappear from sight, but are still working hard at getting you seen to a new audience.

Most importantly, be engaged. Respond to comments you receive, like other people's posts and write comments for feedback. Don't just write to people that are famous and have millions of followers, rather, support the people who support you.

YouTube

YouTube is also an extremely powerful way to reach a wider audience. Not so long ago, getting on TV was almost impossible. Now we live in an age where we can have our own channel! Yoga teachers need to make the most of this, in my opinion! I discovered the power of YouTube for myself when a student of mine was inspired by something I'd taught him in class, so made a video on his channel about it. Both him and his wife had been using YouTube as a successful marketing tool to launch several businesses and then gave me the QVCA formula that I included earlier in the book. What I loved about their approach was that they didn't see YouTube as a marketing tool. For them it was a way of adding value into the community. Their philosophy was you should never try to sell to anyone. Just adding value is enough, because through that people will want to support you for helping them.

Once I realised this I started having fun with my channel. I just wanted to create great content and I wanted to see lots of people progressing. The result was that my online classes started to sell extremely well and I now earn a passive income off the back of my channel.

Just one word of caution. Don't expect to go viral over night. I used to think that if I upload a video tonight, tomorrow I'd have a thousand views and another thousand the day after that. This was completely naive on my part. YouTube is packed with amazing (and not so amazing) content from thousands of channels. Creating a following takes consistent effort and dedication. This is what puts so many people off in the first few months of running a channel. They don't see it explode and they lose interest. Keep at it! If you have good content that has been curated well, a following will form. The Key? Be patient and consistent!

Overcoming Camera Jitters

I know a lot of teachers who aren't comfortable in front of the camera, so the thought of filming themselves and posting a clip on YouTube is extremely unappealing. When I first started experimenting with videos, I was very scared of being filmed and terrified of what others would think of me, but in my heart I felt it would be a great way to reach more people. So I watched a lot of other teachers on YouTube and mimicked the ones I liked. If I saw a teacher doing a sequence with a nice background, I went all over

London looking for a great spot and created a little sequence to match nice music. If I saw another teacher doing a little instructional video, I would find an authentic theme and do something similar. I never copied content, but I always looked to see what was working, then emulated that. Over time this developed into my own style as my confidence grew. One of my videos was spotted by someone who works for Yoga Download (www.yogadownload.com) in America. They approached me to create content, which has been massively successful and earns me a passive income.

Every teacher has something unique and special to offer. It just takes practice for it to come out and shine through. So if your first 10 or even 20 videos aren't massive successes, don't worry! The fact that you are practicing in front of a camera is a great start and will bring rewards in time. Even if you don't get tangible financial benefits from filming, it will make you a better teacher. After all, you will have the opportunity to look and analyse your technique, hear your vocal pitch, and practice your teaching rhythm. This is extremely valuable!

If you're scared of watching yourself then how can you expect other people to come to your classes to learn from you?! As my mother would say to me, *"get over yourself!"*. She didn't mean this as a derogatory comment, what she meant is, stop being so hung up on being perfect. Use tools like this improve aspects of your teaching and at the same time learn to love how quirky you are. The more you 'own' your quirkiness, the more people will be able to relate to you, and the more they will want to learn from you.

Facebook

Facebook is another great platform to get people excited about you and your brand. I use Facebook so that I can add value to people's lives through my posts. I also use Facebook to post my YouTube videos, promo workshops and retreats and share what I find interesting in the community. It's also a cool way to connect to people more personally as many write to me and express things in personal messages. This is special because few other platforms provide this level of connection.

One day after class a girl came up to me and told me about how she loves my classes but that she struggles to keep her attendance regular because she has to travel for work a lot. I will never forget what she said, *"Celest I miss you so much when I am not in London, but you know I always feel like you are with me. I read your heart warming posts every day on Facebook and Instagram and your pictures inspire me to keep practicing."* This goes to illustrate the power of social media and proves that you can create a sense of soulful connection and build a sense of community via your online presence.

Twitter

I'm not a huge fan of Twitter. I can't keep up with it. It's a relentless machine of text and I also find the set word count per post very limiting. However, it can be useful, once you have a following, to get free stuff. I don't personally utilise this feature enough but I have a friend who has been given festival tickets, a juicer, food for a week and a month driving a new car, all because he said he'd tweet about it to his 3000 followers. Companies are always looking for new ways to get their latest products noticed by the masses and these days corporations don't invest all their marketing budget into old fashioned styles of advertising. Many are now targeting bloggers and people who have a big social media following to push their products to the public.

Another bonus (like Facebook) is that you can add clickable links to each post. This is invaluable for people like us who are running workshops, retreats, selling online content and promoting our other social media platforms.

Fake Followers and Playing Games

It's tempting to want to grow so badly that you start buying fake followers or playing the follow/unfollow game. The follow/unfollow game is where you follow loads of people in the hope that they will follow you back. Then you go back and unfollow all of them, regardless if they showed you the 'follow back' love or not. Buying fake followers can make you appear to be bigger than you are and this can build credibility in the eyes of some people. The bottom line is both strategies can work, but in the process you compromise your integrity and may lose the respect of your community.

I remember once talking to one of my students about social media and I expressed to her that it's a lot of work for growth that is very slow. "Yes" she said, "but you know I can see that you have grown very organically without playing any games. I know a yoga teacher in our community who has followed and unfollowed me four times!" Needless to say this student lost respect for that teacher and the way she handled her social media.

Buying followers can also be painfully obvious when your interaction levels are low. You should be getting around one to three percent of your followers liking your content and about seven percent of the likes should be commenting on the post. If this is consistently not the case it shows that you might have bought followers which looks a little bit tacky and desperate. In some ways I respect you for being a little hustler. But like my dad always says, "sometimes slow is fast and fast is slow."

I follow people who's content I love and unfollow people who's content I don't love. That is my only strategy. I like and comment on other people's posts if they are great and don't if they aren't. I have no agenda. I might be growing more slowly for it, but the fans that I have are true fans who genuinely love me and my posts.

Website Image

Having a good website is an essential marketing tool and demonstrates your level of professionalism. Unfortunately, we live in a very superficial world, and if your website looks amateur or unprofessional, people won't take you seriously. Whenever I stumble across a website that lacks quality and isn't userfriendly I immediately start questioning the credibility of the information and feel frustrated by the clumsy navigation. I'm not alone. Many people will judge you by your website, so make sure you take the time to build a good one.

Having a good website doesn't have to cost an arm and a leg either. I spent a bit more on mine as I felt my time was better spent earning extra money to pay for a professional to do it. That said, there are some awesome WordPress templates (also called themes) out there if you have the time or the inclination to create your website yourself. The most important thing is that the end makes the person browsing curious about you and your services.

The Art of Analytics

Of course, having a website that looks good without anyone actually finding it is like erecting a billboard in the desert. This is where analytics are really important. I used a company to boost my website's SEO and Google rankings. If anyone searches for me, or my company name, my website pops up first. Again this might take a bit of investment but it will be really worth it when you start gaining more private clients. If you know someone who is good with analytics, ask them if you can teach them private yoga in exchange for helping with your website analytics.

Collaboration

A fun way to expand your marketing capacity is to collaborate with other people who are doing exciting things in the yoga community, with whom you resonate. Make a wish list of people you'd love to work with and find ways to make your professional world's collide. This can be beneficial in a few ways. For one thing, you can learn skills from them if they're more experienced than you; And for two, you can double your audience reach by hitting two databases instead of one.

A good example of collaboration in action was when lululemon organised flash mobs in different locations all over London one summer. A few different teachers were picked to lead the mobs and I decided to ask one of them if I could help her promote hers, as the attendance for the other flash mobs had been pretty low (less than 10 people!). She admitted that she'd decided to cancel hers because so many people had said they couldn't make it.

I offered her the option of collaborating with me. I told her my flash mob date and that we should hook up and make something magical happen where we both taught together. She was totally keen on this idea and we set up a Facebook page together and started spreading the word. Over 50 people turned up at our flash mob on the day! Which was a much bigger crowd than either of us would have gathered individually.

Since then I have collaborated on all sorts of things, including a Physiotherapy for Yoga Teachers course; my health blog on YouTube; capoeira workshops; weekend retreats; physiotherapy training; and even Instagram photos. These were all awesome opportunities to learn, grow and take what I do to a new level, with the support of other teachers in the yoga community.

Business Admin

Whether or not you're into self-promotion, social media and marketing is a necessary part of running any business nowadays. So although being on the mat teaching is where the magic happens, like every job, there are aspects to being a yoga teacher that aren't as fun as others and you need to embrace those too.

As my mom always used to tell me: *"Celest, there is no perfect job. Every job has an element of repetition and things that you will not enjoy. Even famous singers have to sing the same song, over and over again, and every time they have to find passion and enthusiasm to make it sound great. You have to do the same. If there are elements of your work you don't like, find the passion behind what you do to make what you do great!"* I have always held onto these words and when the time came for me to promote myself, they served me well. I've invested countless hours researching what made all this social media and marketing stuff work for me. I didn't want to do it, but I did it because it was a stepping-stone to other great opportunities. And in my case, it's definitely paid off.

Chapter 3

EXPERT

Hanging Out in Pincha and Smiling

Congratulations my fellow yoga superhero you are now reaching the peak pose of your journey. This is the time when we want to start positioning ourselves as an expert in our field. Getting *Pincha Myaurasana* right takes some positioning and lots of practice. Similarly, as a yoga teacher you will have to work on your positioning over time and with persistence. Being a more advanced student in yoga is not only about mastering arm balances and inversions, it's also about understanding your own mind on and off the mat. As your career in teaching starts to take off, don't just aim for the fame. I think the rewards in your career lie in connecting to the people who love your style in a very genuine way. And on top of that, you have the skills to help take them to a higher level physically and mentally. Now we have to get your superhero skills to the next level! By positioning yourself as an expert in your field.

Sharing Your Expertise

The definition of expert in the dictionary is, "A person that is very knowledgeable about or skilful in a particular area." My definition: "an expert is being known in your community as a bad ass who knows their shit". If someone needs some guidance, they come to you! This definition denotes that one needs to have invested time and effort in acquiring either information about a topic or practiced a skill repeatedly so as to have the ability to perform it at a high level. In my opinion, true experts do one more thing: they share their expertise openly and add value to the wider industry so that their knowledge can positively impact as many people as possible. For example, the teachers that run charity workshops, offer free content on their websites and post complimentary classes on YouTube, are the ones who thrive the most.

What Goes Around Comes Around

After I'd been teaching for a few years, but still wasn't making enough money to make ends meet, I decided to film some yoga classes and sell them on my website. In my head it was easy. I'd film a series of classes, get a friend to edit them, upload them and boom! I'd be a millionaire overnight. I forged ahead with my plan and filmed some sequences, and sat next to my friend for hours editing the content. My first wake up call was learning how long it really takes to shoot and edit content. I was buzzing with excitement the day the content went live on my website and was convinced I would soon be sipping cocktails, swinging in a hammock somewhere in the Caribbean celebrating my online success.

Of course, that didn't happen. The content sat there for weeks with only about four or five sales. Then a friend of mine told me, "Hey Celest, you know a lot of people give content away. Why don't you do that?" I thought, "What an idiotic thing to do. I'm spending my precious time making something so that I can make a bit of money, not so people can see this stuff free." But a few months later I started creating content on YouTube, free value for all to see. And this made a massive difference in attracting opportunities. I was giving away free content and this slowly started positioning me as an expert in my field. Creating months of free content showed I knew a thing or two, had some skill, and was worth offering opportunities to. That was when everything shifted for me. My first break was being asked to teach for Yoga Download, an online platform that sells yoga content. I actually did feel like a superhero flying out to the USA to shoot for their platform. I'm still by no means massive, and yet my teaching is reaching a far wider, international audience. Can you imagine the potential that lies ahead of us all if we can find a way to share what we know for more people to see?

There Is No Substitute for Hard Work

Sometimes the most well-known teachers aren't the ones with all the knowledge, but are the ones willing to work harder and smarter to raise their profiles. I like to call this 'the hustle'. By the time my career started to take off I started attracting a great deal of opportunities purely because I was willing to work long hours to grow my brand and become the best I could be. There is a lack of longevity in the yoga industry and plenty of competition. The great thing about competition is that it forces me to constantly think about how I can become the very best version of myself as a teacher and means there is no excuses for complacency.

Being known for the right reasons has always been high on my priority list. By the time I started getting professional recognition for my work, I had already experimented with various styles of yoga and teaching formats, and had a strong social media following that was attracting attention from all over the world. "Bamboo!" my friend Hari would often say to me. "You plant that stuff and it can take up to seven years of watering and attention before you see it break through the ground. Then, it grows like a weed." He was right. I had been working hard on refining my craft as a teacher and spent endless hours building my profile on social media and before I finally started seeing bamboo shoots sprout.

Finding a Mentor

Finding a mentor can be challenging, but can also be an extremely important step to progressing in your career. If you're a coach, get a coach. Likewise, if you're a yoga teacher, attend other teachers' classes, find a teacher that inspires you and ask them for guidance. A mentor can be someone you pay for advice, or someone who just hangs out with you out of the goodness of their heart to see someone else progressing in the direction of their dreams.

I've personally never had a teacher from the yoga world give me the help and guidance I asked for, but I've had very successful business people offer me their expertise. One of my clients was a CEO of a multimillion-dollar company and he taught me about positioning. One of my students gave me invaluable insights about social media strategies. Lululemon spent time helping me with goal setting. My parents told me to take risks. My brother taught me to laugh at the world when it wasn't going your way. My friend Marketa showed me how to get the most out of the least amount of time. And finally, my friend Hari, taught me a great deal about the mind and how to get the best out of it. There have been plenty of others and I credit my professional success to all of the mentors that have helped guide me along the way.

As I mentioned earlier, I spend a lot of time helping other teachers. I used to do it for free and never asked for anything in return. But these days, because I'm so busy I exchange mentoring for help with various admin related tasks. This way we both get to grow.

Pay It Forward

I truly believe that the more you give in life, the more you get in return, so I tend to offer free advice to as many people as possible. Ask yourself if in the future, once you have 'made it', will you be happy to offer free advice or will you prefer to be compensated in some way for your time? The answer to this question will give you an idea of what you are prepared to do now. If you think you'll be someone who will charge, then you need to be prepared to pay for a mentor now. However, if you're not prepared to pay for a mentor now, then make sure that you're prepared to 'pay-it-forward' further down the line. As the motivational speaker Zig Ziglar once said: *"You can have everything in life you want, if you just help enough other people get what they want."* Giving freely is the single most important step that I've learnt in my growth as a yoga teacher. I encourage you to do the same.

Being Professional

It might seem like the next section is self-explanatory, but you'd be surprised at how many people don't raise the bar when it comes to their level of professionalism. Small things make a world of difference. Many teachers are great at teaching yoga but if they aren't professional this sticks out in people's minds over and above anything else. Although worrying about what other people think of you is a waste of time and energy, word-of-mouth is the most effective form of advertising, so make sure that if people are talking about you, it's about how great you are, not about how dirty your fingernails were or how you are late for every class. Here are a few important points to bear in mind:

• Always turn up to work showered, clean and neat. I use natural deodorants because I want to avoid chemicals, so I shower twice a day. Nothing is worse than a sweaty, smelly yoga teacher!

• Always brush your teeth twice a day and don't eat smelly foods like garlic food before your classes. Remember you go very close to people when doing adjustments and it's extremely rude to hover over someone if you smell of coffee or onions. Be respectful, it's their class after all.

• Turn up at least five minutes before your class is due to start. Being consistently late is unforgivable. If you know that you are not great at time-management make yourself leave the house 30 minutes before the appropriate time to leave. It's far better to be too early for class than it is to be late. I always strive to be at least five minutes early so that if anyone wants to ask me a question, I'm available. Likewise, I structure my day so that I have time to take questions at the end too. You'll be amazed at how much people appreciate having access to you as a teacher. They'll support you again and again if you give them just a little bit of your time.

Teaching an Outstanding Class

By the time my full-time teaching career had started, I had already been training as a devoted capoeira student for eight years. I loved it! But even more than that, I was fascinated by the skill and leadership qualities of our teacher. He was a young man in his 30's, but he conducted himself as if he was much older and demanded we treat him as such. We were happy to oblige because we loved training with him. He was inspiring and we all believed that a little bit of his magic would somehow rub off on us.

As my teaching career began I was painfully aware that after my classes, I didn't have people come up to me and express how much they had enjoyed the session. I also only had a very small group of students that would return to my sessions class after class. This bothered me. My capoeira teacher was very popular. He sometimes crammed over 70 people, mostly regulars, in one session and always had lots of people wanting to speak to him after class to express their gratitude. I couldn't work out what I needed to do to make this happen in my career.

At first, when I started expressing this to my friends, I was told that my ego had to step aside. But I couldn't shake it. Was it my ego that needed external validation? I decided that this was part of it, but what I also realised was that this was a symptom of being a remarkable teacher. I wanted to be outstanding. I wanted to deliver classes that would leave people inspired to live better lives. I wanted students to return week after week because I was helping them in some way.

Fake It Till You Make it

The desire to improve got me studying. I started noticing what my favourite teachers in various disciplines did in class that made them so popular. I noticed their body language, the structure of the class, how they interacted with students, the tone of their voice. I absorbed everything I thought was a part of the reason they were doing well and I began to practice, what they call in NLP (neuro-linguistic programming) "act as if". I began to imagine that this quality or personality trait was a part of me. I would talk more loudly and with greater articulation, I moved more confidently, I began pausing the class when the students weren't doing things exactly how I wanted. Some of these things worked well, others were a huge failure.

In the end I discovered that the things which inspired the people in my class more than anything was being unapologetically myself. When you emulate other confident people some of that naturally rubs off on you. My self-confidence was in a healthy place and this greater sense of self-belief helped me to be more ME. This was when the biggest shift in my career started to take place. I was taking big risks. My classes were not 'traditional' anymore. I loved the poses but my favourite thing to do was talk about self-development topics that had inspired me. Each week I looked for something new that would inspire me, and I would use that at the start of my class as the 'meditation'. I also felt that the way we broke postures down in capoeira was fantastic for improving, but in yoga this wasn't the norm.

I began incorporating my passions or 'U.S.P's' (unique selling points) into my classes and soon they were buzzing with more and more people. All my classes were selling out, and there was always a waiting list of up to 10 people lining up in the hope someone wouldn't show. Even my off-peak public classes became so popular the studio where I teach had to move me into a bigger room to accommodate the numbers.

"Acting as if" is basically a way to refine your superhero skills. You have to figure out who you are as a teacher along the way and then maximise those skills full out when you are teaching. With time what you'll discover is that you BEING YOU is your biggest superhero skill.

Refining Your Style

Developing your own style takes time, but there are a few things that can make the transition from beginner to seasoned teacher a little bit easier. As a new teacher there is a great deal of information that you need to get your head around – you are concentrating on the safety of the students, their form, your instruction, the pace, their abilities, offering alternatives, the list goes on and on – so having a basic plan in mind of what I wanted to cover in the class was really useful when I first began. It took the pressure off so I didn't have to worry about which pose comes next. For example, at the start of each week I prepare a sequence or two for my 'Vinyasa Flow' classes so I already have them in mind.

Every class is obviously a little different depending on the skill level of the class. Some will be more advanced, some less, and learning how to spontaneously tweak the class you prepared so that everyone can progress in their own way and at their own pace is a great skill to hone. This has been often referred to as 'reading the room'. Reading the room is a skill that takes time to develop. You might even get to the point where you don't need to prepare anything.

For me, even though I can use my intuition now to teach on the fly, I still like to prepare. This helps me to step out of my head and into the class room, making me far more attentive to the needs of my students.

Catering to All Skill Levels

Dealing with different skill levels is an essential part of building a loyal following. I found I needed to learn how to make the class hard enough so that everyone was challenged, but if anyone was uncomfortable with doing a certain pose, injured, or new to yoga, then I taught alternatives to keep everyone in the class engaged and entertained. This tip however should be applied with some discretion. There are some people that will attend your class who will demand a lot of your time and energy and you will exhaust yourself running around in an attempt to please everyone. On some level you need to assert your authority as a teacher and stick to your guns. Nowadays I offer alternatives and modifications, but if there is someone doing their own thing and ignoring me I leave them to their own devices, occasionally intervening with a little encouragement or support.

Please Yourself, Not the Masses

Similarly, there might be people that'll demand your attention but are always complaining. At the start of my career I did my utmost to please everyone and failed miserably. Some liked the heat up, others down, some people enjoyed the music I played, others preferred silence. As I kept working on pleasing the masses my love for teaching started waning. I realised the students were in control, and were dictating what my classes should and shouldn't involve.

This was the moment I took back my authority. The room temperature was going to be slightly higher and the music was going to be upbeat, loud and fun. I adopted the attitude that if you didn't like it then that's ok because I honestly didn't mind if you didn't come back. I would openly say, "Guys if you don't like this please don't come back!" People would laugh when I said this. Most people are silently impressed with this level of confidence. I call it my super power!

Pace Yourself

Teaching can be extremely tiring. I used to think it was okay to do four or five classes every day. After all, other people were working 12-hour shifts, so why couldn't I do five classes? Well, teaching is a whole new way of using your mind and body and it's demanding on so many levels. Coupled with the travel time between classes and the interaction with students before and after, your energy starts waning and giving your best in every class becomes harder and harder. It's really important not to have a short-term mentality when seeing yourself as a teacher.

For a while when I first started teaching, I kept thinking of how great my pay cheque was going to be for all the extra hours I was putting in. What I didn't bargain for however, was being completely exhausted for 50% of my schedule. As a consequence, I started teaching some really average classes and subsequently, started losing clients and opportunities. When I cut my classes back to three a day, occasionally teaching four and giving myself a day off, my teaching was fresh every class. I was genuinely excited to be there and this translated into packed classes and more private clients who stayed on my books for years. Further down the line I had the confidence to raise my fees and scale classes back to a maximum of two a day. This meant I had time to develop my self practice, work on creating a more sustainable business model while earning the same amount.

Being a yoga teacher often means accepting a reduced income and making ends meet can be a challenge in the beginning, but try your best to see the bigger picture. If you can shine in every class, it won't be long before you're making a great living doing what you love.

My Golden Teaching Tips

I have been teaching yoga for six years now (2015). In that time I have gained some invaluable insights and learnt some key lessons that I feel passionate about passing onto new teachers who are trying to break into the industry. As with all of the advice in this book, don't use the below suggestions if you feel they won't be an authentic extension of who you are as a person. I'm simply sharing what helped accelerate my career, but everyone is different. So take what resonates with you and ignore anything that doesn't. Nothing is written in stone.

• Talk about your personal journey in class to inspire your students. Whenever I teach something that is challenging to the students, I always talk about my struggle to attain that aspect of the practice. I speak about when I fell over, landed flat on my face and burst out into hysterical laughter.

• Don't be too dogmatic. The best way to inspire your students to be the best they can be, is to lead by example. In my own way I work hard at being healthy to inspire people to also embrace a healthy lifestyle. I also like to buy really cool vegan shoes and bags from my favourite websites to prove that being cruelty free is easy and super stylish. I stay away from preaching to people about how cruel the fur industry is, because although it is true, it just makes people defensive (trust me, I tried).

• Use scientific evidence to back up some of the esoteric elements of the class. I love to briefly quote studies I've read that prove how important it is to meditate, express gratitude, breathe deeply and any other benefits I'm highlighting. This makes the class all-inclusive so that the people who already know how beneficial these aspects are, are reminded that they are on the right path. To the people who feel these elements are a bit 'airy fairy', they get a chance to expand their awareness of yoga's wider lessons and value.

• Get the less advanced students to demonstrate postures in class. One of the best ways to raise the enthusiasm of a student is to point out the things they are doing to make the impossible, possible. One of my students was particularly tight in his legs from years of playing football. However, after only four months of doing yoga, he managed to get up into a headstand from wide legs. I got him to demonstrate this to the class and he lit up like a Christmas tree with excitement. That week I had seven other relatively new students attempt postures they never thought they could do and they all succeeded.

• Challenge the students to do new things that they think they can't by breaking the postures down into manageable steps. Don't be scared of teaching poses that are tricky in your class. If the students don't want to do them, they simply won't. But I guarantee that the majority of the students will be thrilled to be given something to work towards.

• Work on your voice. When I first started teaching I realised that my voice was quite high-pitched and I spoke really fast. So I raised my awareness and learnt to use the deeper aspects of my voice. I also make a point of pausing and speaking more slowly (I still struggle with this one). It's really important that your voice is smooth and continuous, but at the same time engaging by using a tonal variety.

Remember that with yoga we tend to use our auditory capacity more than any other sense to get through the class. If you don't have a strong voice or a rhythm that is easy to listen to, get a vocal coach. I did this and I never looked back. I'm sure I still have a lot to learn, but where I am now compared to where I was is miles apart and the coaching has made a big difference to my teaching. On the flip side, don't alter your voice to sound like someone other than yourself or you won't sound natural. If you change your voice, tonality or pitch to sound like someone else you'll sound strange. Strike a balance.

• Get the students to work in partners. Whenever I feel the energy in the room is dipping, for whatever reason, I get the students to work in two's or threes. This gets them to progress on their own practice, when we're working on more advanced postures, because they have to assist their partners and give advice on how to improve. When they are working on helping their partners relax or stretch out, they are building on their body awareness inadvertently. My favourite reason to get people to work in two's is that it builds a sense of community in the classroom. So many people live lonely lives where there is little or no connection between each other, especially in a city like London. Getting them to partner up with people they might not know, get's them to meet the people they share yoga with week after week.

Never become complacent. Constantly ask yourself, *"How can I improve?"* Your brain will go off in search of the answer and will, on a very deep unconscious level, keep moving you forward. This is a strategy I use a lot. I'm not someone who is naturally good at things the first time and have had to work really hard to progress in my craft. When I first started teaching, I taught some classes where students walked out of the room they hated my class so much. This is all part of the process and you have to be prepared to go through this humbling, sometimes humiliating, right of passage in your teaching career. At the risk of repeating myself, I'll say again, get comfortable with not being perfect. Using the yardstick of perfection as a measure of success will only cause you stress, since no class is ever 'perfect'. However, as long as you're learning, you are moving in the right direction.

Chapter 4

ECONOMICS

Time to Stretch

Making ends meet as a yoga teacher can be a challenge. It's not that you don't make enough money to pay your bills when you're working, but what happens when you take a holiday or get sick? Because the bills never stop, many yoga teachers don't stop working either. They work non-stop until they burn out, get injured or stop enjoying teaching. They forget the passion that inspired them to become yoga teachers because they are just too tired. Many also cease to maintain their own practice. This is not going to happen to you yoga superhero because I am here to teach you how to stretch your long term vision, budget, and earnings. Just like you know the value of stretching in your own practice, so one also has to spend time stretching your self into a new income bracket.

The Harsh Reality

The reality of being a yoga teacher is that you will also be working anti-social hours. When all of your friends are having fun on the weekend, you'll be teaching. Evenings, teaching. Early mornings, teaching. There is no question that being a yoga teacher can be extremely lonely at times. The small amount of free time you'll have available to run errands and socialise will be during the day when everyone else is at work. During your 'time off', you'll be catching up on admin – writing invoices, posting on social media, planning marketing strategies, doing self-practice. There is a lot to do behind the scenes and many up-and-coming superhero's get to the point where they feel overwhelmed and throw in the towel. I'm not being overly negative telling you these details, these facts are the honest reality of having the best job in the world.

Taking The Plunge

Perhaps you are a newly qualified teacher who is teaching a little on the side, but you can't bring yourself to leave your current job even though you hate it and are desperate to leave. The first thing you need to do is create a savings account as a backup plan. Then work out how much money you need to survive. Ask local teachers what the least amount of money you will get paid per class would be if you were starting out in gyms and community centres. Most teachers say they need between 12 to 15 classes per week to get by. Once you have worked this out you can set a realistic goal of working to attain at least a third of these classes while still in your current employment.

Most of your classes will be in the mornings, evenings and weekends. You will have a short period of time where you will be working really hard, because all of your time off will be spent teaching. Use this period of time to save all of the money you make from teaching. Set a date where you will hand in your notice to your boss, and stick to it!

You will come up with millions of reasons why leaving the safety and security of your job is a bad idea but it's important that you stick to your decision and make the change. Alternatively, you might be able to work out some kind of part-time or job-sharing scenario that requires you to only work some of the week. Either way, with some savings in the bank the pressure will be lighter and you will be able to search for more classes without feeling too much financial pressure. Once you have around seven regular classes the rest will come quickly. You'll be surprised how quickly.

Quick Task:

Write all the pro's and con's of staying in your current role. Write all the pro's and con's of doing yoga full time. This exercise is designed to get you to see the reality of the situation. Being a yoga teacher is actually quite tough. If you can see the full picture and still want to do it, then nothing will stand in your way!

Budgeting & Bookkeeping

Creating and sticking to a budget and keeping an eye on your bookkeeping are extremely important aspects of running a successful yoga business. Your income will be coming in from various places so if you don't keep track of your paperwork, it will become tricky to stay on top of your admin. So draw up a flow chart weekly and make notes of how much you earned from each venue or person. Also keep the receipts of what you spent so you get a clear picture of where your money is going. Set up a 'sister' account that makes it easy to drop 20% off all your earnings for your tax. Regular savings for your tax bill is essential. Also, saving for a rainy day is important too. Set up as many extra 'sister' accounts as you wish, so that you can easily put a percentage of your savings away as soon as you get paid. The most effect form of saving is to set up a direct debit that automatically deducts money from your salary every month. That way you won't miss the extra money as you never had it's luxury in the first place. As your income increases, make sure you keep amending how much you deduct from your tax and keep increasing the amount you put away for savings.

Accounting

For the first two years of my teaching career I did a self-assessment as a self-employed individual. Then in my third year, I set up a limited company and became the director. The company then paid me a salary every month. To do this you need to hire an accountant. I found that the money I spent on the accountant was well worth it. It meant that I had someone with the appropriate knowledge guiding me. I also paid the least amount of tax that I owed. Make sure you pay your taxes correctly but don't pay any more than you need to. That's why a good accountant is essential. They'll guide you correctly and keep both you and the taxman happy.

If I could go back and do it again I would take the latter option of registering as a company from the start. It works out far better and was much more economical for me. Plus, it gets the correct infrastructure in place for you to grow and expand your business faster. As you gain a higher profile and earn money from multiple income streams, you will need an accountant anyway. Finding an accountant from the beginning means you can build a relationship with them and can see if they are the right person to support you as you grow.

To find an accountant, reach out to your mentors or put a message on Facebook asking if anyone has any recommendations. Show them your accounts and ask them if a limited company is the way to go. It was for me, but with any advice you are given, always take the time to do your own research and make an educated decision.

Creating a Passive Income

After falling into the trap of becoming a slave to my demanding teaching schedule, I decided to come up with a plan that would help me create a 'passive income', so that I could continue making money without being physically present. Because while running workshops, retreats, and teaching private clients are all great ways to generate extra income, they still require a huge time and energy investment. If you limit yourself to only getting paid for being present, you are living hand-to-mouth and will never be free. The key is to get away from exchanging your time for money. To do this it's essential to think creatively 'outside the box'. Find something you can create once and earn from repeatedly. For example, my love of performing was always one of my super powers. So I channelled that skill into the camera and started earning a supplementary, passive income from that. By creating passive income streams you can avoid the yoga 'rat race'.

Creating a Savings Plan

As a yoga teacher you don't have someone automatically paying money into a pension account for you. You also don't get paid if you don't work. Which is why you must have some savings up your sleeve! As yoga teachers we are taught to live in the moment and very rarely do we stop and think about our financial future. But without planning we could end up being very sorry in the future.

I know many teachers are on a spiritual path and might take offence to how strongly I feel about this topic, but I have witnessed the devastating results of poor financial planning first-hand. When I was studying physiotherapy I had the great privilege of going out into the community and working in the Elderly Care sector. It was painfully obvious if the patients we were working with didn't have the foresight to put money away for their future. Many were living off the state pension, which is a dismally low amount. Survival is all these poor people can afford, and as a direct result of that, their quality of life is dramatically affected with many falling into depression.

For this reason, I encourage you to create a savings

account and be diligent about putting 10 to 20% of your income away as soon as you get paid. When I give this advice to people I often receive resistance. The biggest excuse is that they can't afford to do that, and that if they did they wouldn't make ends meet. However according to a well-known phenomenon psychologists call the 'Parksinon's Law', "the demand upon a resource tends to expand to match the supply of the resource" – so no matter what you earn you will always raise your level of expenses and your standard of living to the point where you feel you cannot afford to put money away. In other words, the more you earn, the more you spend.

Which is why, no matter how little you're earning, it is extremely important to put aside a percentage of your earnings regularly and never touch it. Turn saving into your super power. Initially this will be challenging, but after a while you will make clever adjustments to your spending to make saving possible. If 20% is too much, start with what you can. Even if it's only one percent, to start with. You might think that one percent is not worth it, but the most important thing is to get you into the mindset and habit of putting money away and never touching it. Once you start saving you will find that the reserve of money in your bank account creates a great sense of independence and confidence. It will also help you in tough times, if you lose classes, clients, becomes sick, or incur any other unexpected expenses.

Investing

In addition to saving you should learn about investing. I haven't got any formal training to be a financial advisor, and because I am young, I don't have enough life experience to share advice that is sound, proven and tested. However, I can say one thing with certainty: money that is just sitting in a bank account or under a mattress loses value over time.

Although I'm not an expert, I've sought out investment advice from friends and family members that have the experience in this field. What I have learned is that investments fall into two categories: high risk or low risk. According to the experts, splitting your money into a few different pieces is the way to go. One piece should remain in a bank account untouched; another should be placed in a low-risk investment option that grows slowly but steadily with time; the other piece should be placed in a high-risk investment that has the potential to grow quickly. Whatever you do, make sure you don't invest all of your life savings in one place. The more places your money is, the safer it will be. Don't put all of your eggs in one basket!

Some resources that can help educate you about investment strategies is the book *'Money: Master the Game'* by Tony Robbins and David Bach's audio programme, *'The Automatic Millionaire'*. There are many good quality resources out there, but these two are my favourites. They are both pitched to an American audience, so you might have to get some advice from friends and family that have more experience in international investments, but ultimately you need to be educated enough to take your own personal risks. The main thing to take from this section of the book is, INVEST! Don't sit on your money. Take some risks. Play it safe. Learning about this game is an important step for your future.

The Power of Financial Freedom

In sharing all of this advice, you may think I've forgotten the true meaning of yoga, "Aparigraha" (non-possessiveness, non-grasping or non-greediness), because I'm overly focused on making money. Maybe I am, but in my heart I really love being a yoga teacher and I don't want to have to stop because I can't afford to pay for my water and lights. I had to take a step back, look at what I was doing and find creative ways to use my passion for teaching to get me to a point where I could teach two or three classes a day, instead of five or six, and still cover my bills and save up for a rainy day.

Having long-term financial goals isn't superficial. I'm not giving you the above advice because I want you to become a money hungry millionaire. I'm telling these things because taking control of your finances can greatly improve the quality of your life in the short and long-term future.

Chapter 5

ENERGY

The Savasana of Success

The thing about being a superhero is you are often in 'giving mode'. To sustain that output of energy you need to self invest. That means leading by example, and being a living illustration of the positive mental, physical, emotional and spiritual benefits of yoga. Be living proof that yoga gives you super powers! After all, who's going to attend the classes of a tired, stressed out teacher who walks into class with a hangover, smelling of cigarette smoke whilst drinking an energy drink?

On a practical level, when you don't work, you don't get paid. So staying healthy is essential to your survival as a yoga teacher. Take the following advice if you feel it'll work for you. My health suffered a lot when I started teaching so these tips helped me overcome extreme fatigue. But I appreciate that we are all different and therefore it's important to do your own research too. Remember, being fanatical about anything is the worst thing you can do for your health. So just do your best!

Alkalise to Energise

Whether you're managing your timetable efficiently or not, the demands on you as a teacher will stack up and your energy levels will be tested. In addition to classes, you will be writing articles, doing self-practice, running workshops, organising retreats, presenting, doing social media. The list goes on and on and it is extremely important to keep your energy at its highest level.

When I first started teaching I remember being so exhausted that I couldn't get through my evening classes without taking a nap during the day. I used this strategy for a long time until I came across the book, 'The PH Miracle' by Dr Robert O Young. This book changed my life. It taught me the reason I did not have enough energy to make it through the day was that my body was overly acidic and in an attempt to get it back to a state of alkalinity I had to drastically change my diet.

In a nutshell, the book explains that 80% of your diet needs to consist of alkalising foods and the other 20% can be more acidic in nature. Quick chemistry lesson: the pH scale is a measure of how alkaline or acidic something is. It ranges from 0 (very acidic) to 14 (very alkaline). Too much acidity in the system creates havoc – tiredness, illness and disease in the body. However it takes much more alkalinity to neutralise acid. Hence you need to take in more alkaline-based foods.

Every different part of your body has a different pH number. But the river of life that runs through you is set at 7.365 (very mildly alkaline). It will always stay there; if it didn't, you would die. But, in order for blood to remain at 7.365 it has to work really hard if you keep putting acidic food in your system. It will in fact, draw resources from elsewhere to keep you safe and your blood at 7.365.

Foods with the highest alkalinity are vegetables (especially greens), tomatoes and avocados. Lemons, even though they are acidic fruits, have a strong alkalising effect on the body. So I always squeeze fresh lemon juice into my water bottle. You can also invest in a water ionizer, which is a machine that alkalises normal tap water. You can set it from as low as ph 2 (acidic) all the way up to pH 12 (alkaline). I drink water set at pH 9.5 and this has had a miraculous effect on my health and energy levels. Water ionizer's aren't cheap, so a more cost-effective way of alkalising your water is to squeeze lemon juice in your water, buy an alkaline water filter jug, and make sure your diet is as alkaline as possible. One great online resource that gives great alkaline dietary advice is Energise For Life www.energiseforlife.com.

Drink Water

If you're not drinking lots of water already then it's really important that you make it a priority. Water is needed in every single cell of your body, helping them function more efficiently and keeping your toxin levels low. Traditionally, most recommendations call for 1.5 litres a day. However, this is not really enough. According to Iranian doctor, Dr Batmanghelidj, who has studied water intensively and used it to heal illness in people, people should drink around half their body weight in ounces per day. For example, if you are 140 lb (10 stones or 63.5kg), you would need to be drinking around 70 ounces of water or two litres a day. That's just for normal functioning. If you use your body a lot, like yoga teachers do, then you'd need to increase this. Some people suggest that drinking three to four litres a day is even better for you and I personally subscribe to this practice. You'll be amazed at the difference in your mind and body as soon as you increase your water consumption.

Obviously there is a thing as too much water – especially if it creates an imbalance in the body's salt levels – but since most people are chronically dehydrated (and don't even realise it!), this is extremely rare. Let your body's natural intuition guide you on this and increase your intake gradually over a number of weeks.

Cut Out the Bad Stuff

To create more energy and be the best you can be as a teacher you need to take one simple step: cut out things that harm the body.

Sugar

Remove sugar from your diet. Although this is extremely challenging because sugar is hidden in a lot of packaged foods nowadays, there is no good reason to eat refined sugar. Although our cells need glucose (simple sugars) for energy, high levels of fructose (fruit sugar) and sucrose (cane sugar) can disrupt your blood's natural glucose levels and damage cells in the pancreas, which in turn negatively affects your insulin supply and can lead to diabetes. According to recent statistics released by the

World Health Organization (www.who.int) an estimated 1.5 million deaths were directly caused by diabetes in 2012 and by 2030 it is projected that diabetes will be the seventh leading cause of death.

Although these figures are alarming, many cases of diabetes can be resolved and reversed through diet changes. There are many reports of patients with type-2 diabetes reducing and eventually eliminating their need for insulin by simply changing their diets to plant-based wholefoods and cutting out –sugar. The film 'Simply Raw: Reversing Diabetes in 30 days' is an extremely insightful film about people with type-1 diabetes who reverse the course of the disease through diet, without pharmaceutical medication. Definitely worth watching to see how powerful food can be in a short space of time.

Alcohol

Many people feel that it's acceptable to have alcohol on a daily basis. Lots of people I know relax by drinking a glass of wine every evening. They don't get drunk or lose control; they simply use alcohol to ease daily stress. Although this is socially acceptable, it is damaging to your health because no matter how small the amount, alcohol is a poison. It interferes with the mechanism that regulates the water levels in the body, causing dehydration, and has a detrimental effect on the body's largest organ – the liver. One of the liver's many functions is to filter and clean your blood, and since alcohol remains in your body until it is processed (by the liver) once it has entered your bloodstream, you make the liver work twice as hard when you drink. In fact, it takes about one hour for your liver to break down one unit of alcohol. Also, when alcohol reaches the liver, it produces a toxic enzyme called acetaldehyde, which causes inflammation and can damage liver cells. Think of alcohol as black sludge being poured into your body's purification tank.

What's more, alcohol has the ability to break the blood-brain barrier (BBB). The BBB is a highly selective 'diffusion barrier' that separates the brain from the circulatory system and protects the central nervous system (CNS) from potentially harmful chemicals. In other words, it is the brain's inbuilt 'security system', which allows the entry of essential nutrients while blocking other damaging substances. Unfortunately, the brain doesn't recognise alcohol as harmful, so alcohol can pass through the BBB, reaching brain cells and neurons directly, which then interferes with the brain's communication pathways.

These disruptions can change mood and behaviour, making it harder to think clearly and move with coordination. Drinking too much also weakens your immune system, making you much more susceptible to colds and flus. None of which are good for your health or for your yoga teaching career. I do enjoy an occasional drink, but because I don't drink alcohol regularly, I find it only takes one or two to get me tipsy. So that means a night out on the town is much cheaper than it once was. I've also not had a cold or flu for four years. Please keep having fun! Don't cut alcohol out of your life completely, but be aware of the amount you consume and how that might effect you.

Coffee

Ok now I recommend you sit down. Because your whole world is about to come crashing down. Yes, am going to tell you what you already know. Coffee is not your friend. Although coffee gives you a short-term boost, it over-stimulates the adrenal glands, causing high levels of acidity in the blood. Consequently, the body has to work extremely hard to regulate your cortisol levels and maintain the delicate balance in the blood. In the process it uses up large amounts of energy which is the reason your energy crashes in the afternoon, no matter how much coffee you drank in the morning. Have you ever gone a day without coffee? Noticed what happens? You get the worst headache of your life. Why? Because your body is addicted to it, so going without your coffee fix is like a mini version of a heroin addict going cold turkey. Detoxing from your daily coffee habit and switching to something healthier like green tea is something every coffee addict should try. I promise you'll feel better in the long run. Have fun experimenting with macha lattes, yum!

Smoking

With the amount of information available today proving all of the negative effects smoking has on your health (lung cancer, decreased bone density, skin wrinkles, emphysema and optic nerve damage, to name a few!), it seems crazy to smoke cigarettes. Tobacco smoke contains more than 7,000 chemicals, all of which go directly into your bloodstream and into your organs. Not only does smoking compromise the immune system, making smokers more likely to have respiratory infections, but it doubles your risk of developing rheumatoid arthritis. It also makes your breath, skin, hair and clothes smell like a chimney, which will be noticed by your students. If you're a smoker and you want to quit, get support and find a way to give up. Allen Carr's 'Easy Way to Stop Smoking program' is meant to be a great method. Also, give hypnosis a go. I use hypnosis for almost everything and the results have been incredible. If all else fails, girls remember, smoking gives you wrinkles. And boys, it makes you impotent. Need I say more?

Gluten

A few years back my stomach started to act up. I didn't think anything of it at the time, but when it was clear it wasn't just a passing phase I started to experiment with cutting various things out of my diet to see what the trigger might be. There was a definite shift when I stopped eating gluten and dairy, but I don't think I was strict enough with it. My stomach was always up and down and I had extreme fatigue. The biggest wake up call was when my hair started falling out in bunches. It turns out gluten was affecting the way my gut absorbs nutrients. Now I know not everyone is as sensitive as I am, but the more research I have done the more I realise that gluten is something worth avoiding.

One book I read, named Gut by Giulia Enders, explained it perfectly. Remember the old saying, "everything in moderation!" Well the issue with gluten is it's in almost everything. Also over the past 20 years, it's gone through a huge process of genetic modification. The body therefore doesn't recognise the gluten protein and simply cannot cope with the huge doses it has to process.

Screen Time

My friend Tony became very unwell with extreme adrenal fatigue and had to take months off from his job as a TV presenter to get back to good health. When he recovered he started a podcast all about energy (Zestology), where he interviewed a lot of clever people in the field about what tips and strategies they had to share that could help people improve their health and gain more energy. One of the themes that keeps repeating itself on his podcast is the effect that digital screens can have on a person's energy levels. I decided to give this a try for myself.

Each day I would give my energy a rating out of five-

five was feeling great and one was tired. I mentally tracked my energy levels in this way over the course of a few weeks and I concluded that, without a shadow of a doubt, my energy levels were at their highest when I spent prolonged periods of time away from screens. I then took it a step further and I would notice how screen time affected my classes. Now, I KNOW that if I am on my computer a lot before I teach a class, the quality of the class will be affected. So I have to take a break from all technology before I teach. Everyone is different, so it's worth experimenting to see what works for you.

Add in Good Stuff
Sleep

Without a doubt, sleep is the most important part of maintaining a healthy mind and body. Imagine taking your car to the garage to get polished and cleaned while a mechanic looks at the engine and ensures every part of the engine is in the best condition. This is what sleep does for your human body. It helps the body repair itself. As a yoga teacher you need to make sure that you are getting great quality sleep so you can keep teaching outstanding classes, day after day. Without it your classes will suffer. You just won't be able to inspire your students if your batteries aren't fully charged.

When I first started teaching I wasn't looking after my health properly which meant I needed to take long afternoon naps to give me the energy I needed to get through my evening classes. These days I tend to go for short 20 to 30 minute power naps (although not nearly as frequently as when I needed those long afternoon sleeps), and strongly advocate getting a power nap whenever possible. They will keep you sharp as a razor in your classes. Having said all that, many people can't nap in the day as it throws off their sleep patterns or makes them groggy in the afternoon. As ever, let your body's intuition guide you on this.

The best way to get a good night's sleep is to establish a regular sleep pattern. Make sure that when you get home at night your routine supports getting you into a state relaxed enough to fall asleep. Avoid jumping on your computer or watching television (and especially watching the news!) right before bedtime. What you do first thing in the morning and last thing at night have a massive impact on the health of your mind, as your subconscious is most susceptible to information at these times. I often listen to inspirational audios in the morning while I'm getting ready; and in the evening I meditate. Sometimes if I'm really tired from a long day of teaching, I practice yoga nidra (yogic sleep). Do whatever works for you.

As many of you know, melatonin is your sleep hormone produced by the pineal glad in the brain. It's also a powerful antioxidant which helps fight cancer cells in your body. The pineal glad needs darkness to produce melatonin, however these days with bright lights and devices the pineal glad turns off the melatonin production every time blue light hits the retina of the eye. The more hours of darkness the pineal glad has to produce melatonin the better. But if you check your phone in the middle of the night to see the time, your melatonin production goes down to zero! Thankfully some clever people have produced some cool things to help us out. To eliminate the blue light from my lap top I downloaded an application called F.lux. And no that's not a spelling error, it's F.lux! Remember the dot when you are researching this super cool invention. F.lux works on a timer and turns your screen amber when it's time for bed.

I also bought some blue light blocker glasses. These are great for when I finish work late and head home on the tube. Sometimes my house mate is watching TV or has the lights on, then I wear them around the house. If he's not around I light candles everywhere and get ready for bed in semi-darkness to start stimulating my melatonin production. You might think I'm a little nutcase, walking around with blue-light blocker glasses on at night, but it's made me feel so good I just have to keep this crazy habit up.

Detoxing & Cleansing

No matter how healthy you are, your body is always working hard to keep toxins at a manageable level. Going on a detox helps your body remove excessive waste that builds up and can make you feel run down or sick. The first detox I ever did was a three-day fast in Thailand, followed by a one-month detox at home. This didn't involve fasting but I did cut out all sugar, including fruit, most grains, alcohol, tea and coffee. I ate lots of fresh vegetables with a little tofu combined in the most radical, imaginative ways. Since then my health has never been better.

If you want to pinpoint specific areas of your health that are in need for improvement, I recommend doing a live blood analysis. This involves going to see someone who will look at your blood under a high-powered microscope. The health of your blood really dictates the health of your body. It is the river of life running through you. It's fascinating seeing all your cells, the blood plasma and even the immune system working away. What is scary is you also see yeast, microforms, parasites and even food floating around in your blood. These little 'creatures' deplete the nutrients in your system and decrease the immune system's efficiency.

The best way to combat these is to eat healthy nourishing food that they dislike. Microforms can only survive on sugar, yeast and processed foods. If you eat fresh vegetables, lentils, beans, nuts, seeds, millet, rice, sorghum, amaranth, quinoa and tofu (to name just a few), combined in inventive ways, the microforms have no choice but to perish. They simply cannot survive when you switch to a plant-based, wholefood diet. You on the other hand will thrive! You'll be amazed at how great you're going to feel and how good you're going to look.

Taking a Yoga Break

As a teacher you do your utmost to maintain some type of a regular self-practice, yet sometimes when you're tired, overwhelmed and time-starved the last thing you feel like doing is climbing on your mat to practice yoga. Personally, I find practicing to my fullest potential by myself challenging, so at four times a week I find a class to attend. I also really enjoy doing activities that don't have anything to do with yoga.

Taking a break from yoga allows you to create the headspace to find new inspiration to share when you're teaching. I found going to capoeira, gymnastics, CrossFit, dance classes, Pilates and kickboxing kept me inspired to progress in my practice in new ways. That said, the activity doesn't have to be other forms of exercise. It could be singing lessons, painting or even joining a book club. It's really important that you give to yourself so that you have enough to give as a teacher. Sleep in, go for a massage, get your nails done. Even if you're a little tight on cash in the short-term, the energy you'll gain with fill you with fresh enthusiasm for what you do, which will shine through and help you grow in your field in the long run. Stay focused on your goals and work hard, but stop and smell the roses along the way.

Doing something interesting outside of the yoga world helps to maintain a sense of balance and keeps your feet on the ground. Many teachers I meet that do nothing but yoga lose the ability to relate to a variety or people because they spend so much of their time with yogi's. Branch out and use the opportunity to grow the yoga community by being an inspirational person that steps outside of the box and makes an effort to expand as an individual.

Meditation

Maintaining a healthy work/life balance is an essential part of being a good yoga teacher. Looking after yourself is part of your job. Especially looking after your mind. One of the ways I stay sane is through meditation. I'm aware that meditation is not for everyone, even if you're a yoga teacher. So my advice is to explore lots of different types of meditation so that you can find the right fit for you.

When I went to India to do my teacher training I met several people that raved about their experiences doing Vipassana meditation. I didn't know what this was, but soon learned that it was a type of meditation that involves complete silence for 10 days and about eight hours of mediation per day. When these people told me about this I thought they had completely lost their minds. "Who would do such a strange thing?" I thought. Then, due to a series of crazy circumstances towards the end of my journey I found myself in Bangalore, sitting in an ashram meditating for hours and not talking. That's right, I was doing the crazy Vipassana thing I had laughed about before. This experience was probably one of the hardest things I ever did in my entire life. But it was also one of the best.

Vipassana taught me, on an experiential level, the nature of impermanence. It also gave me the chance to learn how to deal with life in a less reactive way. I felt a great sense of calm when I left and still to this day kept up a regular meditation practice. However, the strategies taught in Vipassana didn't work for me in my life back home. I kept up the practice of sitting still and breathing, but sometimes I did positive visualisations, gratitude meditations, self-love mantras, etc. I mixed it up. Sometimes I even found I was too tired physically to sit and meditate, so I started to lie down and do guided mediations like Yoga Nidra or hypnosis.

My favourite hypnosis tracks are from Paul McKenna. When I first started to teach I found myself being very nervous and overly anxious. Needless to say, this had a negative impact on my confidence. So my friend recommended I try the confidence hypnosis by Mr McKenna. I was skeptical at first but kept using it to give me a perfectly timed 30-minute power nap. Months later I started noticing how I would say positive things to myself when I was about to teach. Even if the class didn't go quite as well as I would have liked, I kept telling myself that I am great at what I do and I can learn from my mistakes. Off the back of this my classes started to flourish. At the time I couldn't quite work out where this new super power had come from but later when I managed to stay awake through the hypnosis tape I realised that it was the script from the recording.

Visualisations were not only great for my yoga career, but they helped me feel less anxious about the future. I would take the first few moments to just focus my breath and relax in a seated, up right position. Then I would allow my mind to see all the things that wanted to manifest in my life. I let myself walk through this vision as if it had already happened. Believe it or not, some of the things I visualised did come true. Others again did not. That's ok! I think positive visualisations should be practiced by everyone.

When I am really tired and my mind can't settle my favourite meditation is the gratitude meditation. In this meditation I take the time to think about everything in my life that I am grateful for. I literally will say the words in my mind, "I am grateful for my eyes. I am grateful for my family. I am grateful for…" I just keep going and going and going. There is never a bad time to do this meditation. It has the most powerful, positive effect on my mind and I am a huge advocate of doing it regularly.

Whichever type of meditation you choose, make sure it's something that adds to your life in a positive way, makes you a better person, and helps you deal constructively with the pressures of life.

Psychological Health

The biggest hurdle I had to overcome in my own teaching was learning to control my own mind. As each new class would begin my mind would start reeling. Negative thoughts would dominate, telling me how stupid I sounded. The most common thought was that everyone in the class was hating the session and couldn't wait for it to end. I believed that I knew what these people were thinking purely based just on their facial expressions. When I looked around the room, if anyone didn't look completely engaged and present, I would take that as a sign that they thought I was awful. The downside to this was that my thinking was shaping my reality. You can't think these thoughts and teach a great class at the same time. Negative thoughts effect your performance, massively. So I learnt the art of controlling my mind.

After my trip to India, I had a solid meditation practice. I'd spent the majority of my time there in ashrams and I felt like my mind was more peaceful and centred than it had ever been. But teaching seemed to magnify whatever wild-mindedness was still present. Just like alcoholics anonymous, encourages people to first acknowledge they have a problem before it can be addressed, this was my first step too. I realised that my lack of performance as a teacher was my own imaginary creation, secondary to believing that the people present were not enjoying the class. It was hard to get over this. But over time, whenever I realised I was spiralling into negativity, I would stop and take a step back and would make myself think a positive thought. It wasn't an overnight shift, but slowly over time I could see that the quality of my classes were improving and with that my following grew too.

Assess the Company You Keep

As entrepreneur, author and motivational speaker Jim Rohn once said, "You are the average of the five people you spend the most time with." With this in mind, ask yourself, 'Who do I want to become or emulate?' Personally, I like to hang around with positive, happy, healthy people; People who strive for their goals through the good and bad times. Your closest peers have an incredible influence on you and its important to make sure you are surrounding yourself with people who use their super powers for great things in this world. This will inspire you and lift you up, especially when doubt comes knocking.

Action Point:

Make a list of the people you currently spend the most time with. Make a list of their positive and negative traits and assess for yourself if these people are supporting you in the best way possible. This can be a challenging area for some people, especially if they've been friends for years. The truth is that we all have different paths to travel in life and some people are more suited to your lifelong journey than others.

If there are some people on the list that have negative traits that leave you feeling energetically depleted or drained, it is time to do some boundary setting. This might not mean cutting these people out of your life completely, especially if they are family. It simply gives you the chance to reevaluate how much time you currently spend with them, and in what capacity. How can you continue to support them as a friend without decreasing your own energy levels? On the flip side, increase your exposure to your other superhero's, those people who lift your spirits, walk their talk and bring good into this world.

Chapter 6

EVOLVE

Let's Om

Wow my yoga superhero, what a journey we have been on. This is by no means the end! If anything, just like the Om at the end of a yoga class doesn't mean you stop being a yogi, but rather that you keep living the teachings of yoga on and off the mat, in the same way, with your yoga business, you have to constantly search out ways to grow and expand your super powers.

There are some unique and special people in this world whose calling in life is to develop their spiritual practice and being a yoga teacher is one way they can fuel this burning desire. Other yoga teachers, such as myself, love being a yoga teacher and want to turn it into a viable business. In addition to teaching, I want to publish this book, teach workshops all over the world and make video downloads so people can do yoga anywhere, anytime. I want to earn money from my downloads while I sleep. So that one day if I have children, I will still be earning enough money to live a comfortable life and help support my family while I'm not physically out there teaching.

To achieve my goals I've had to stand out from the myriad of incredible yoga teachers out there. I had to build my personal and professional confidence from a grassroots level, creating a signature style and brand identity along the way, as well as slowly building a tribe of followers who want to be a part of my vision and community. I credit some of the success I've experienced to my journey in personal development. Through various books, courses, teachers and self-growth authors, I picked up various 'tools' that have helped me to excel in my teaching. This chapter is me openly and honestly talking about what worked for me. I'd like to encourage you to add to this chapter in your journal and share what you have found worked for you with others one day. I'd love to hear what resources have pushed you ahead in your career and made you the superhero of your story.

The Power of a Smile

My first introduction to personal development was when I was 12 and my mother gave me a book called, 'How to Win Friends and Influence People', by Dale Carnegie. This book contains lots of relevant lessons for teachers and I am grateful everyday to my mum for giving it to me at an age when it could shape my personality in a lasting way. A lot of factors have contributed to my success in life, but the lessons I learned from this book lies right near the top. One of those lessons, as simple and lame as it may seem, was the power of smiling. As Dale Carnegie says, "The expression one wears on one's face is far more important than the clothes one wears on one's back."

Although I had ugly braces on my teeth at the time, I made it my mission to walk around with a smile on my face. At first it felt a little forced but then I found my mind finding things to smile about. The best part is, smiling is contagious. When you smile at someone else, mirror neurons are activated in their brain that create microscopic muscle movements that mimic the smile on your face. Research has shown that smiling releases serotonin – a neurotransmitter that produces feelings of happiness and wellbeing. So now, not only are you feeling happy but you've just made someone else feel happy too. It's contagious. As a yoga teacher use your smile whenever you feel like it when you're teaching. For me, being natural and smiling as often as I felt like it has made me seem more approachable. It's helped me build strong bonds with my students and loyal fans.

The 'State Change' Technique

Another great source of personal development, education, motivation and inspiration is seminars. One of the standout seminars that helped propel my career to the next level was a four-day course led by seasoned American peak performance coach, Anthony Robbins, called 'Unleash the Power Within'. I attended the course when I was about 18 months into full-time teaching and was extremely doubtful that all the effort I was putting into my work would be fruitful. A big part of me felt very scared and uneasy about the future and I was carrying some serious self-limiting beliefs. To say that the seminar turned my life around is an understatement. It gave me a huge kick up the butt and helped me turn around my state of mind from a place of deep self-doubt to self-empowerment. He gave us lots of little tips and tricks that can be applied in the classroom to make you a better teacher.

One that I use regularly was the process that deals with creating a 'state change'. Something I am frequently asked is, "how do you cope when you're having a bad day?" In my opinion, if you're unwell or sad when you teach, it's not really professional to walk into a class and say, "Guys, if today's class is not that good it's because I'm really tired and having a bad day.'" You may disagree with me, but personally I always maintain a strong sense of professionalism as a teacher, even if inside I don't really feel it. I achieve this by using the 'state change' technique that I was taught in the Anthony Robbins seminar. Here's what this involves:

1. Close your eyes and remember a time in your life when you felt wonderful. You woke up beaming, you felt great, the day flowed and nothing but magic was happening all day long.

2. As the memory comes up, see what you saw and feel what you felt. If you are looking at yourself in your mind's eye as if you were another person, step inside your own body.

3. Remember how you moved, how you were breathing and especially your facial expression.

4. Seeing all those aspects, embody those elements now as you remember this scene.

5. Noticing what emotions come up, allow these emotions to magnify tenfold. You can continue magnifying these emotions as many times and as big as you want.

6. Hold onto all of these feelings and step inside of your body at this moment in time. Come into the present and keeping these emotions in your body.

This simple process is something I use regularly. It's not that I'm faking it, I'm just tapping into another side of who I am. Some people say I can do this because I'm better at this 'stuff'. The truth is, the only difference is that I have been practicing this technique longer and now I only need to do it for a minute to get the desired effect.

How Not Why

Another very important personal development lesson I've learnt over the years is to pay attention to the way I speak to myself. The voice in your head is more powerful than you think and is thankfully in your control. However cultivating a positive internal dialogue takes practice. Most of the time we ask ourselves constant questions. For example: "why did I say that?"; "why am I always late?"; "why can't I get anything right?"; "why do people always let me down?"; and "why I can't I be as successful as so-and-so?" These are examples of negative questions that your mind might be asking, either on a conscious or unconscious level. Very rarely will something positive come from asking these questions, instead they steal your super powers.

They also have a very deep effect on your actions.

Your brain is a bit like Google. If you ask it a question, it will go off and find you the answer. So if you ask it "why am I always late?" Your brain will go off and find all the answers, backing them up with references from the past. "That's just the way you are!"; "You can't help it"; "You have timekeeping issues"; "When you were little you were forced to be on time and now you have a negative association to it." The same goes for questions like, "why do I always mess up in class?" Your brain will think of all the reasons why you are the type of person that always messes up every class.

So how can you reframe this habit and make a positive change? The brain will always ask questions. The trick is to change the questions you ask from a WHY questions to a HOW question. If you are always late ask, "How can I arrange things so that I'll be on time, every time?" Then the brain will go off and get you the answer. "Leave earlier"; "Wake up earlier"; "Organise your bag the day before"; "Plan better." How questions are my way of becoming a superhero when the last thing on earth I feel like doing is being super.

There are a thousand ways to be on time, but your brain will only be given the opportunity to find the answer if you ask the right question. The same goes for the question, "why do I always mess up in class?" Instead you can ask, "How can I teach a class that is wonderful?" The brain then has the opportunity to come up with answers such as "Plan your classes thoroughly"; "Be present by doing a mini meditation before every class"; "Eat enough healthy food every single day"; "Get to know the student's names"; "Play cool music in class". The key is to raise your awareness about what questions are being asked in your mind daily and how you can modify your thinking to give you a chance to really excel in class as the great teacher that you are.

Re-defining Failure

Redefining failure in my head was one of the biggest changes I made in my life and I would say it has contributed to being instrumental in my growing success as a teacher. Many people do something, fail and then feel bad about themselves and stop moving towards their dreams. They feel like they should completely abandon ship and find another path. This is understandable. Failure feels bad. We've been wired to avoid it since we were little. The only problem with being scared of failure is that you never really do anything of value unless you face up to those fears. Living your life in your comfort zone won't bring you the life you dreamed of and you won't access the privilege of helping others.

Failing Forwards

To transcend to a new level, you have to step into the unknown and yes, the possibility of messing up is massive. And yes, the bad news is you probably will. The good news is the more you keep trying and keep failing, the more you will improve over time. Have you heard the expression, "Failing forwards"? Whenever I do things that don't work out how I thought they would, I think of it as one step closer to where I want to be. Learn from the failure and you'll be moving forwards in the right direction.

The Journey is the Destination

Most people base all their self-confidence on the result instead of focusing on the effort they put into the process. If you are guilty of this habit, I encourage you to start focusing on the journey, not the destination. That way your self-confidence is likely to remain consistent and be less at the whims of whether things worked out the way you planned or not. Putting all your focus on the result leads to a total rollercoaster of emotions. Up when things are good, down when things are bad.

Instead, learn the art of equanimity. Become satisfied with every result and instead feel pride for how hard you worked to achieve what you have. Can you remember where you were last year? See in your mind everything you've been through and how far you've come. You are doing extremely well. I know that, because for someone to invest in a book like this you have to have a drive and determination to reach new heights with what you do.

Personally I see every failure as an opportunity to grow and believe if you're not growing you're dying. I never want to stop growing, so if failure gives me the biggest growth then I embrace it with both arms! Most of people's fears are based on what others will think of them. What you have to remember is that what other people think of you is irrelevant. It's what you think of yourself that matters.

Dealing with Rejection

As your career starts taking off you will encounter some criticism along the way. I'd love to tell you that they are just haters and that they don't know what they are talking about, but that won't change the fact that getting negative attention can be hurtful and knock our confidence. When this happens it's really important that you do something called 're-framing'. This is when you think of a situation in a slightly different way to make it serve you. For example, many people in the yoga community criticised me for using social media because they saw it as a superficial medium. So I reframed this to, "social media is a great way to reach more people with my message and help them improve their lives". In this instance I reframed the situation by thinking of rejection or negative feedback as an opportunity to grow. I didn't let those negative people put me down and am so happy I followed my heart and intuition.

It's also important to remember that negative people don't care much about you if you're doing badly because then they have nothing to slate. But if you're doing well people love to poke holes in what you're doing and criticise your methods. Therefore, with that in my mind, whenever I get negative feedback I reframe it and think to myself, "wow, I must be doing really well!" I know that sounds silly, but I never allow harmful comments to upset me. I just smile and see the feedback as an indirect confirmation that I'm doing well.

Setting Goals

Setting solid goals has been the single most important step I've taken to become a successful yoga teacher in my community. I honestly believe the quality of your life is determined by the quality of your focus, so even if you do nothing else I've suggested in this book, I highly recommend you define your goals and diligently write them down.

I learnt this very useful trick from a book entitled 'Goals' by legendary business philosopher, Brian Tracy. One of the exercises he suggests is to write down 10 goals each and every day, for 30 days, without looking back over the goals that you wrote down the day before. The beauty of this process is that it allows you to get clear on what your goals are in the present moment. Yes, they will differ day to day, but as you go through the month, day by day (never looking back at what you wrote the day before), the important ones will keep reappearing and you'll also start getting extremely focused.

Below is a list of some of the goals I wrote down during my 30-day goal-setting challenge.

1. I taught a successful class at the London Om Yoga Show

2. I teach at top London yoga centres such as Triyoga

3. I teach one class a week at the luxury spa, Equinox

4. I have had an article published in Om Magazine

5. I am featuring in lululemon's print advertising

6. I am now a lululemon brand ambassador

An important point of note: I wrote all my goals in the present tense as if I had already achieved them. And guess what? Within that 30-day period and during the weeks following, many of these goals HAD come true! Believe it or not, by listing my goals on paper, lots of awesome things (that were out of my control) began to happen – all helping to elevate my career.

Another great goal-setting resource is Igolu (<u>www.igolu.com</u>) by lululemon, who offer anyone and everyone free downloadable 'vision and goal templates'. Their interactive format means you can either watch online videos and complete assignments independently over four sessions, or go through the process with the support of a certified Igolu leader. The programme is designed to empower you to create the personal legacy you want to leave in the world, and is an extremely helpful way to define your goals and start making them a reality.

Something is Better than Nothing

Along with my professional goals, I also wrote detailed goals for my health and personal life. Many of the things on this list also came true, and the ones that didn't are by no means totally off the cards. Remember, the point isn't to tick off every single goal on your list, the point is to define the goals in the first place and to TAKE ACTION. I know a lot of people that are hesitant about writing goal lists because they're afraid of feeling a sense of failure if they don't achieve them. Let's reframe that mentality. Say you write down 10 goals and only one or two of them come true, then you've still achieved those two goals. Celebrate! Up until then, without them written down, you hadn't achieved anything. Better to have 20% of your goals realised rather than 0%!

After all, as American philosopher Suzy Kassem once said, "Doubt kills more dreams than failure ever will". I still have my whole life to buy a house and start a family. That is the magic of goals. If you miss your deadline for achieving them, you simply set another one. You get to move at your own pace and achieve them when the time is right. You also get to change them. The goals you care about now might change in a few months. Brilliant! Change is a natural progressive part of life. Let your goals embrace change too.

Set Big, Scary, Unrealistic Goals

The key to goal setting is to set big, scary, 'unrealistic' ones. I remember asking my friend once what her goals were and she told me she wanted to go to the cinema and buy her mum flowers. I was shocked, to say the least, and instantly blurted back, "That's not a goal list, it's a 'to-do' list!" She explained that her reason for not setting 'big' goals is that she was afraid they were too unrealistic. "What if they don't come true?" she asked me. I asked her the reverse question, "What if they do?!"

The truth is, many of life's greatest achievements and the world's most life-changing evolutions occur because someone was willing to be unrealistic. As Nelson Mandela once famously said, "It always seems impossible until it is done." People have bent sheets of metal into tubes, which have flown countless people across the globe; We can talk to our families on the other side of the earth on a handheld device with no wires and they sound like they are sitting right next to you; We can access any piece of information on any topic within seconds thanks to network called the internet. All of these achievements began as someone's goal. Someone who was probably told they were being unrealistic by their friends and colleagues. In the moments when fear or doubt holds you back, remember the words of Bon Warn, "If you're going to doubt something, doubt your limits".

Strengths Finder

Another incredible resource that helps you discover your unique strengths and teaches you how to use these to excel in your life is a book called 'Strengths Finder' (www.strengthsfinder.com). Written by bestselling business author, Tom Rath. This book asserts that all too often, our natural talents go untapped because from a young age, we devote more time to fixing our shortcomings and weaknesses, than to developing our strengths. For example, if you struggled with maths growing up, then everyone would spend more time with you doing sums, timetables, multiplication and division. But it is seldom that people invest additional time in helping you reach your full potential in areas in which you thrive.

Strengths Finder includes an extremely thorough online test that assesses every part of your brain to figure out what it is that makes you tick. It then does a detailed analysis of your character – what your strengths are; how people can relate to you; and how you can use these strengths to move forward in your life. I found this immensely helpful. My top strength is positivity. It told me that I was best suited to a job where I get to pick out the positive aspects around me. This made me laugh, as I am constantly looking for even the slightest improvement in the students that attend my classes, and when there is an improvement I get super excited. As well as defining my greatest strength, the book went on to give me tips on ways to capitalise on this quality and gave me some key pieces of advice that not only made a huge amount of sense to me and have since been instrumental in getting people to take me more seriously in my profession.

Strengths Finder also taught me about the down side of having positivity as a top strength. It explained that people often don't take positive people seriously and that many think positive people aren't in touch with the real world. What I loved, was that the book also shared the practical advice on what to do in this situation. The advice it gave was to remind people who feel this way that positive people are not unaware of the negativity that is present in the world, they just choose not to put undue attention on it. This advice was transformational and made a difference when I was dealing with negatively inclined students.

Be Your Own Guru

Above all remember that you are a wise and intelligent person that has had a wealth of experience. Be open to learning from a variety of sources, but never lose the ability to question things and dig deeper. Make up your own mind and then be willing to change what you learned as new information is brought to your attention. In my heart I know there are many well meaning people out there that position themselves as gurus. Someone with all the answers. Ultimately however you are the one with the wisdom to know whether or not to heed the words of another person, book or video. So make an effort to listen to your own internal wisdom.

Conclusion

If you are inspired to be a yoga teacher, then go for it! It's not an easy job. The working hours are long and antisocial, you don't earn great money at the start of your career and there are times when you'll deal with lots of ungrateful people day in and out. Competition for teaching jobs is fierce. People will judge and criticise your teaching style at times, and more than once you'll think, "Why did I get into this?" Despite this, my advice is to persevere. It takes guts to step into the unknown and teach a group of strangers. Yet every single time you walk to the front of the classroom and lead a class through a series of postures, you learn and grow. This growth pushes you to expand as an individual and beyond that, it cultivates your ability to inspire others to expand.

As a yoga teacher you are automatically placed in a position of leadership. Whether you like it or not, people will look to you as their role model, hero and mentor and will often come to you for advice and help. With this in mind, it is really important to think about what it means to be a leader. In my eyes, a leader is someone who does just that – they lead. They are willing to step into the unknown as pioneers, to make sure their followers are safe. They always put their followers needs ahead of their own and ensure that every time the followers have contact with them, they deliver value in a loving way.

Being a leader doesn't mean always knowing the answer or making the right decision. What it does mean is that you help those around you to grow into the best versions of themselves. Sharing what we know is a great gift and privilege that can help others. Your biggest desire should be to create a positive shift in the people who have contact with you. Receiving glory, praise or fame should not be the goal. Humility is a vital aspect of being a good leader. If that stuff comes, embrace it with open arms, but throughout this book I wanted to inspire you to become the superhero of YOUR life. Nobody else's.

I remember talking to a fellow teacher once who was

complaining that there are way too many yoga teachers coming out of teacher trainings and that these people have no idea how tough it's going to be, as there not enough classes for everyone. I totally saw her point and for a brief second, I saw what she was seeing. But then I reframed my perspective to see only the potential. There are eight million people in London. Only a small fraction of them have taken a yoga class. Most people haven't found 'their teacher' (their superhero) because that person hasn't graduated from their teacher training yet. That person could be you reading this book in another part of the world where even fewer people are doing yoga. You have the potential to become the teacher who sheds fresh light on this ancient practice and touches people's lives in a truly unique way.

In my opinion, teaching yoga is an incredibly rewarding job. I believe that yoga is a great tool that helps people realise their potential and see the divinity in each other. Imagine if the whole world could see the divinity in their fellow humans? Imagine how different life would be. Well that is your job as a teacher – to bring people into the present, lead them into a state of higher consciousness, and encourage them to treat each other with more kindness. I only know a few jobs on this earth that carry such a profound responsibility.

The most important thing to remember, my beautiful superhero, is to always be yourself! The beauty of yoga is that it can be your own blank canvas from which you create a work of art. You can create something very special that will touch people in such a small amount of time, yet make big changes that are good for them and all of humanity. I know that you have it in you. Go and shine. Your students are waiting!

Interviews

At the time of authoring this book I was very aware that it only contained my very narrow perspective. So I decided to include interviews from a variety of amazing teachers, asking what their advice would be for you? I had six incredible teachers sharing openly what they know, Chris Chavez, Rachel Brathen, Irene Pappas, Mercedes Nogh, Lesley Fightmaster and Dylan Werner. All I can say is, ENJOY!

Chris Chavez

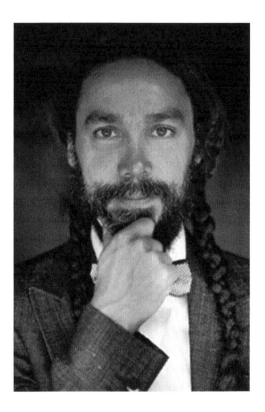

Website: www.chrischavez.com

Chris Chavez is a global yoga teacher based in Istanbul, Turkey. He leads teacher trainings every year through the Chris Chavez School of Yoga and his graduates can be found in locations all over the world. He's also a musician and the Co-owner of Cihangir Yoga Istanbul.

Chris first began the practice of Iyengar yoga in Ireland, where he was touring as a professional musician in the mid 1990s. While traversing the globe playing music and studying various other methods of yoga, Chris imparted the knowledge and the gift of yoga upon everyone he met. In 2001, Chris landed in Los Angeles, California, where he submerged himself into the practice and study of yoga and began to teach and build a community. Certified as an Anusara Instructor between 2006 and 2012, Chris is known for his extensive studies, his vast working knowledge of the mind and body, and his great personable demeanour. Chris is considered to be one of the most sought-after teachers in the world, training thousands of teachers and students every year in North America, Europe, and Asia. Chris's world travels and experiences have made him one of the most down to earth yoga teachers you will ever meet. His teachings are fun, challenging, and spiritually uplifting.

Chris has found the power of practicing and teaching yoga to be an integral part of being a great artist as he continues to maintain a healthy music career and a rockin' yoga practice!

1. What's your story? What led you to become a yoga teacher?

How I became a yoga teacher is a mystery to me even now. It seems that it happened while I was busy making plans to do "other things!"

I first came across yoga while travelling as a professional musician - it was a great grounding element to an otherwise chaotic lifestyle. As I travelled - I'm not sure why - I started to tell everyone I came across that they should do yoga, and if they didn't know how, I would show them the 5 poses that I knew and practiced every day.

Years later, I landed in LA and my house was right across the street from a yoga studio. I practiced at the studio EVERY day and then I would go home and practice for another 2 to 3 hours. Soon I started to invite people to come and practice with me in my living room – I just wanted to share!

When more than 2 people wanted to come, I thought that I need a bigger space. That's when my journey began from sharing yoga in my living room with friends to sharing with thousands of friends a year, worldwide. It has been a crazy and an amazing journey. I am very blessed to be able to share what I love with people who are interested in receiving it!!

2. What advice have you got for newly qualified teachers to become great, inspiring teachers in their community?

SHARE! Don't wait to get a teaching job at a studio!!!
GET OUT THERE AND SHARE!!!

In the beginning, you will need to create your own opportunities to share your teachings and you can do that anywhere!!!!!

Your first students will be your family and friends and friends of friends. Basically, your first students will be people who never thought about doing yoga but are keen to give it a try - because it's YOU!

This is where you become GREAT!

By working with people who have never done yoga and by motivating them and keeping them inspired, this is where you learn to tap into the best of who you are. By starting like this, you learn what it means to communicate and just be yourself in a loving and caring way. If you can do it with these students, you can do it anywhere!!!

Once you have developed yourself, you will feel the need to teach at a studio to validate yourself as a teacher. If it comes it comes and if not, keep doing your thing!

3. Have you got any advice on the business aspect of being a yoga teacher?

Charge appropriately for your service! AND be willing to give your time freely when it's needed (balance here is key). As a trained yoga teacher you have invested a lot of time and money to acquire the skills to teach. So, like any other profession, don't be afraid to charge for what you are offering.

That being said, be willing to give of yourself freely when it is truly needed. There will be situations and people who will cross your path who are in need of your skills and talents but do not have the means to pay you. In these moments, give freely and see it as your opportunity to learn something from the person in front of you. The gratitude that you will receive from someone who you have helped is priceless! By helping them, know that you are helping yourself!

4. Have you got anything you'd like to share - any words of inspiration, about your teaching journey that can benefit a new teacher?

The path to being a great teacher is truly found in you just being yourself! I know, it sounds over the top "yogic", but it's true! When you speak from your own experiences and your words are fuelled by your own desire to share and help others, your students will feel that and they will trust you! The trust they give to you is precious, so treat it with respect.

Also, know that there is no formula and there is no easy way. If you want to be a successful teacher (in whatever way that means to you), you have to do the work!!!! So, GET STARTED NOW! LOVE :))

Rachel Brathen

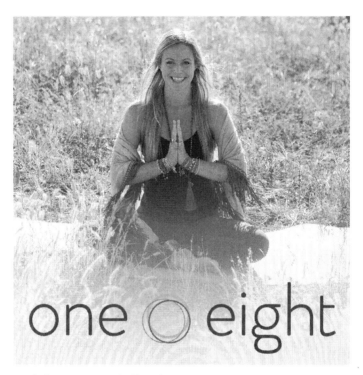

Website: www.rachelbrathen.com,

www.oneoeight.tv, www.sgtpeppersfriends.com

Instagram: @yoga_girl, @oneoeight.tv,

@109world, @sgtpeppersfriends

Swedish native Rachel Brathen is a New York Times best-selling author, motivational speaker and international yoga teacher residing in Aruba. After graduating school in Stockholm she traveled to Costa Rica and it was here that she found the joy of incorporating yoga into her everyday life. Deepening her yoga practice and also taking her first steps towards teaching, she ended up moving to Central America where she spent years exploring the intricate studies of yoga and spirituality. After moving to Aruba early 2010 she started teaching yoga full time on this Caribbean island. Her classes are a dynamic Vinyasa Flow practice, integrating alignment, core work, and breathing techniques with basic poses and creative sequencing. With close to two million followers on social media, Brathen shares snapshots of her life with the world every day and constantly travels the globe to connect with her community.

Rachel recently released her first book, "Yoga Girl", now available worldwide. Part self-help and part memoir, YOGA GIRL is an inspirational and vibrant look at the adventure that took her from her hometown in Sweden to the jungles of Costa Rica and finally to the paradise island in the Caribbean that she now calls home. In YOGA GIRL, she gives readers an in-depth look at her journey from her self-destructive teenage years to the bohemian and beautiful life she's built through yoga and meditation in Aruba today.

1. What led you to become a yoga teacher?

I was very much into yoga and one day I was in class and found myself thinking, if I was leading this class I would do this or that differently. When class was over I thought why not give it a try? I have always wanted to inspire people to be the best version of themselves.

2. What advice have you got for newly qualified teachers to become great, inspiring teachers in their community?

To do the best that they can to find their own voice, to teach from where they are, from their own heart and to not try to aspire to be anyone else.

3. Have you got any advice on the business aspect of being a yoga teacher?

You have to put yourself out there and not be scared to go after what you want. If you want big classes and to teach at big studios you have to try and ask, and do what you can to make the connections that you need to make and take the active steps to get there.

4. Have you got anything you'd like to share, any words of inspiration, about your teaching journey?

When I first started teaching, I felt I needed to be this special type of teacher who was a little outside of who I really was and I didn't really feel the passion. Now, I teach from what I know, which is who I am - It's easy and the passion is there. This means my classes are going to be a little funkier with music, people falling, all that good stuff!

Irene Pappas

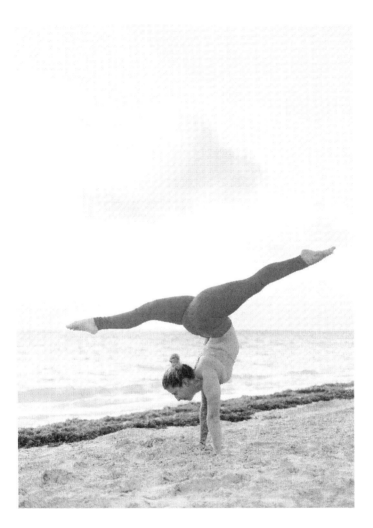

Website: www.fitqueenirene.com

Instagram: fitqueenirene

Irene's love for yoga is contagious. She began practicing in 2012 and immediately knew she had found her path. When she did her first 200 hour teacher training she did not intend to teach right away, but she soon realized that sharing yoga with others was her purpose.

As a lover of movement, Irene is passionate about her practice. She practices both Ashtanga and Rocket yoga, as she enjoys both a traditional practice as well as a spontaneous one. Not only does she practice yoga but she studies with hand balancers, circus performers, and contortionists to expand her own knowledge and explore the capabilities of her body.

After experiencing a life changing wrist injury last year Irene has redefined her yoga practice in many ways, placing more emphasis on a strong foundation and finding gratitude for her body with or without advanced asana. She still enjoys intense practice but has learned to value meditation and pranayama even more, and focuses on sharing this part of her journey with her students.

1. What led you to become a yoga teacher?

When I was 21 I helped my sister open a clothing store, but I knew it wasn't my calling. I was lost and wasn't sure what direction to take my life in. I was beginning to discover my passion for health and fitness but only once I found yoga did I realize what I had been missing all along. When I took my first 200 hour teacher training I honestly did not intend to teach yoga, at least not right away. I wanted to learn more for my own practice, so that I could have a deeper understanding of it. Once I finished my teacher training I subbed a few classes for friends, and I immediately knew I had found my purpose in life. Sharing yoga brought me so much joy and fulfilment, I became a full time yoga instructor and haven't looked back since.

2. What advice have you got for newly qualified teachers to become great, inspiring teachers in their community?

Practice. Many teachers immediately submerge themselves into teaching full time, which is great, but can also be taxing. I would say make sure you remember why you loved yoga in the first place, and never lose that. One of the reasons why students come back to my classes is because I am always teaching new things, as I am always practicing new things myself. And it is not about perfection, whether you are the student or the teacher it is all simply practice.

3. Have you got any advice on the business aspect of being a yoga teacher?

Figure out what makes you different, and continue to move in that direction. Yoga and business can often make for blurred lines, so it is important to stay true to yourself while still promoting yourself in a positive way. Don't be afraid to sell yourself, as long as you do it from a place of integrity and love.

4. Have you got anything you'd like to share, any words of inspiration, about your teaching journey?

I am still at the beginning of my journey as a yoga teacher, and even as a yoga student. No matter how "advanced" your asana practice may become it is so important to stay humble. The practice of yoga can be both a physical and mental journey, but I try to stay grounded and focus on the spiritual aspect.

Mercedes Nogh

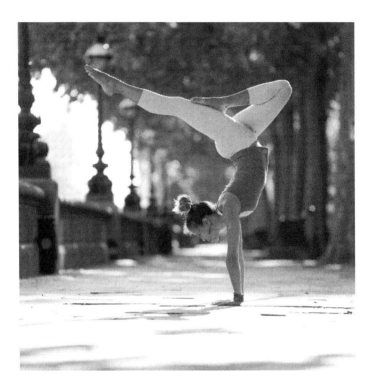

Website: www.mercedesyoga.com, www.yeotown.com

Flow yoga mama to two baby yoginis and wife to an amazing guy, Mercedes Sieff (nee Ngoh) is one of the UK's happiest and most creative Vinyasa Flow yoga instructors. Born in Ottawa, Canada, she spent most of her life studying creative movement and its use as a form of self-expression and spiritual exploration. It was during her time living in California and working in the entertainment industry that she began to study yoga.

As her studies and passion for yoga grew steadily more intense, Mercedes gradually moved into teaching. Having studied various forms of yoga, the primary style she now teaches is Vinyasa Flow. Most of her studies over the past decade have been in California where she has completed different certifications under many recognised teachers including the lovely Shiva Rea.

In 2010 she co-founded the award winning health retreat Yeotown located in North Devon. She is a proud ambassador for lululemon athletica and Manduka and runs weekly vinyasa flow yoga classes, yoga teacher training modules and retreats both locally at Yeotown and abroad throughout the year. Mercedes has been featured on ITV1, BBC Radio and in publications such as Tatler, The Sunday Times , YogaJournal, OM Magazine, Harpers Bazaar and Yoga Magazine. She is a lifestyle and health blogger for the Huffington Post in addition to contributing articles to Mind Body Green, Elephant Journal and Om Magazine. Her latest venture is a juice bar in Marylebone, which will be an extension to her health retreat in Devon.

1. What's your story? What led you to become a yoga teacher?

There was not one particular thing per se that happened that led me to become a teacher. I practiced for years while living in California and as my studies became more intense my interest gradually turned towards sharing the things I was learning with others. When I moved to

London the yoga scene was so different from what I had been part of in LA and there was practically no Vinyasa Flow yoga classes that quite effortlessly and organically I began teaching a lot. I think there was a void that needed to be filled and people were really keen to learn a different style of yoga that was fluid and creative yet powerful and effective.

2. What advice have you got for newly qualified teachers to become great, inspiring teachers in their community?

If you want to inspire others you need to keep inspiring yourself. Often a new teachers' personal practice can suffer when they first start teaching as they sometimes begin to neglect their own studies and practice. Students will be inspired by someone who is curious, passionate and teaches with love and from their heart and for that to happen, a regular practice needs to be in place where you take the time to keep the love affair with yoga alive.

3. Have you got any advice on the business aspect of being a yoga teacher?

I noticed the graduates from my teacher trainings that got on studio timetables and started teaching the most right away were not always the most talented ones nor the ones with the strongest physical practice, but rather they were the ones who put themselves out there and 'hustled' so to speak. They knocked on studio doors, got in touch with gyms, put flyers up around town, put on their own classes in church halls, got a website together - essentially they made their teaching intentions known and taught whenever, wherever, and to whomever as much as they could.

4. Have you got anything you'd like to share, any words of inspiration, about your teaching journey that can benefit a new teacher?

Keep going to other teachers, other classes. Keep studying, keep learning. I don't believe in this 'One voice, one teacher' concept but rather to me yoga is such a rich tradition, science, art etc. that it commands many voices, perspectives, interpretations, minds and hearts to do it justice and you can learn so many different things from so many different people from all backgrounds and traditions. I think that well known African saying "it takes a village" to raise a child is applicable in the way that "it takes a village" to make a great yoga teacher!

Lesley Flightmaster

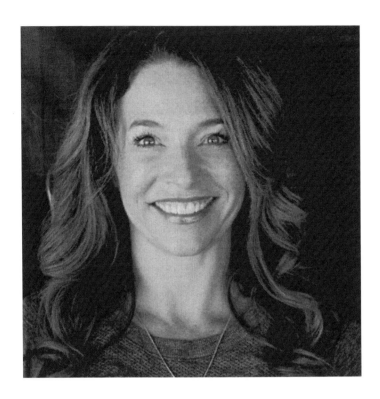

Website: www.fightmasteryoga.com

Youtube: Fightmaster Yoga

My name is Lesley and I love yoga. I have a husband and two boys. Sometimes my sons, Indy and Stone attempt yoga, but their main thing is Brazilian Jiujitsu. My husband Duke is the one behind the camera (making my YouTube videos).

I lead a breath-focused, alignment based class that combines my deep love of movement with the practice of yoga. I believe that the transformational gift of yoga should be available to as many people at possible.

I am a certified instructor registered with Yoga Alliance. I earned my 200-hour certificate through YogaWorks in 2006 and went on to complete my 300-hour training to become E-RYT 500 certified. I'm currently on the faculty of the YogaWorks teacher training department. I lead 200-hour certification programs and teach in the 300 hour program. I would describe my teaching style as an infusion of meditative and flowing Vinyasa classes with yoga philosophy, concise technical alignment, and some heart-felt humour.

1. What's your story? What led you to become a yoga teacher?

I struggled with alcohol abuse when I was younger. I stopped drinking a long time ago, but I still had a lot of anxiety. I wanted to be able to meditate but I couldn't sit still for anything! I began practicing because I had heard that asana practice is a great preparation for meditation. I loved it! I was able to completely relax in Savasana and it was the only time my head was quiet, in the beginning. I had some amazing teachers in San Francisco, where my practice began. I admired them so much and when I moved to southern CA, I decided I wanted to try to inspire others the way they had inspired me.

2. What advice have you got for newly qualified teachers to become great, inspiring teachers in their community?

I think the best advice I can give to new teachers is to keep their practice. It's hard to keep a daily practice because we get so busy, but it's the only way we can continue to learn and inspire others.

3. Have you got any advice on the business aspect of being a yoga teacher?

It's honestly been difficult to make a living, but if you love it, you have to do it no matter what!

4. Have you got anything you'd like to share, any words of inspiration, about your teaching journey that can benefit a new teacher?

I have always looked at teaching as a way to help others to be happier. I know how transformational the practice is and I want to share it with as many people as possible.

Dylan Werner

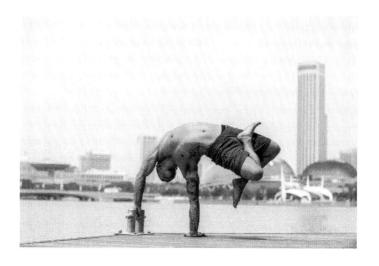

Website: www.dylanwerneryoga.com

Instagram: @dylanwerneryoga

Dylan Werner is an inversion and arm balance master and is regarded as one of the world leaders in yoga strength training and body weight movement. Dylan is a diverse teacher, able to bring the most advanced concepts of yoga and movement to anyone at any level. With a background in wrestling, rock climbing, martial arts, health and fitness, Dylan found yoga to be a culmination of everything he loves. He was first introduced to yoga through his martial arts training. Dylan started teaching yoga in 2011 after 10 years of advanced movement training. While his practice appears very physical, he believes it's only a tool to discover yourself, find clarity, peace, presence and meditation.

1. What's your story? What led you to become a yoga teacher?

I actually never wanted to be a yoga teacher. I loved being a student and had a career as a firefighter/paramedic. I took a teacher training just to support my girlfriend who wanted to be a yoga teacher. During the training, I really fell in love with teaching so I decided to teach part time for fun at my local studio a few days a week. A few years later, I got laid off from the fire department. I wasn't happy with my job so I decided to switch careers. I moved to LA and started teaching full time.

2. What advice have you got for newly qualified teachers to become great, inspiring teachers in their community?

Teach what you love and teach your practice. Don't try to be like anyone else. People go to teachers that are passionate about there practice and what they teach. If you teach from your heart, if you are transparent in your journey, students will be attracted to that. What makes a great teacher is who you are, not your sequencing and not your cues.

3. Have you got any advice on the business aspect of being a yoga teacher?

Be consistent. Be dedicated. Work hard and say yes to every opportunity that comes along. Eventually you'll get to a place where you can pick and choose but until then teach as much as you can wherever you can to whoever you can.

4. Have you got anything you'd like to share, any words of inspiration, about your teaching journey that can benefit a new teacher?

If you want to be a good teacher, you have to have a good self practice! All a yoga teacher does is share their practice. If you don't have a practice to share, you have nothing to teach. Also experience as many teachers as you can and learn everything you can.

Acknowledgements

(Little letters to the people that have helped me along the way)

Chris Chaves, Rachel Brathen, Irene Pappas, Mercedes Nogh, Lesley Fightmaster and Dylan Werner, I don't even know how to thank you guys. I wrote to so many teachers, and as you can imagine, many didn't respond or they turned me down. Thank you for having the humility to help me and for enriching the content of this book.

Mom and Dad, you guys have shaped me. I'm crazy, loud and I struggle with academic things, but none of that matters when I'm with you, because you love me just how I am. I think that unconditional love and support is what has made me so determined to strive for my dreams. I love you both so much.

Albe, thank you for making me see the funny side of life. I never have a straight face around you - it's always creased up laughing. Thank you for helping add more humour and light heartedness into this work. I appreciate the time you spent with me dearly.

Hari, without you this book would not exist. Thank you for giving me the idea, inspiration and self belief to make it happen. This book is filled with all the great things you have taught me during our time together and I will always be grateful for that. For anyone reading this, make sure you look up Hari Kalymnios for inspiration on how to be super human.

Nataliya, your eye for detail and design was instrumental in this journey. I know you have high standards, so when you liked the book you put me at ease. Thank you for taking the time to look at my work and give me advice. Thank you for believing in what we created.

Rebecca, my beautiful editor. Thank you for editing this while a little person was growing inside you. I am happy we met, not just because it has helped me refine my work and improve it, but because you are such a beautiful person. www.thewellnessnomad.com

Jane, thank you for your tireless edit of the first draft. I know the book is very different now to what it once was, but without your keen eyes looking at it the first time my confidence to send it out would have been far less. You're an amazing person and I have always admired you. Keep being you - you're one of the wittiest, loveliest people I've ever met.

Jahan, I sometimes try and imagine where I would be without your support. And I know in my heart I wouldn't be very far. You deserve all the greatness life has to offer, and more! Together I feel like anything is possible. I owe you everything. Thank you so so much!

Nattaka, your purity, kindness and generosity are mind blowing. I can't thank you enough for being a part of my life and helping me grow. You believed in me when not even I believed in me! You're a great friend.

John, you light me up. Thank you for helping me realise the value in rest and consistent training with no compromise. Thank you for supporting me through the highs and lows of life. I'll make an audiobook just for you!

Lotte, thank you for helping me with the edit and using your talents to support me. It's people like you that have helped me get to where I am. I can't wait to see you teaching everywhere!

To the all the yoga teachers who had enough faith in me to ask me to be their mentor; thank you! The moments we shared over teas and coffees were the first beginnings of this book, before it became a tangible creation. Without all of you it wouldn't exist.

DISCLAIMER AND/OR LEGAL NOTICES: Every effort has been made to accurately represent this book and it's potential. Results vary with every individual, and your results may or may not be different from those depicted. No promises, guarantees or warranties, whether stated or implied, have been made that you will produce any specific result from this book. Your efforts are individual and unique, and may vary from those shown. Your success depends on your efforts, background and motivation.

The material in this publication is provided for educational and informational purposes only and is not intended as medical advice. The information contained in this book should not be used to diagnose or treat any illness, metabolic disorder, disease or health problem. Always consult your physician or health care provider before beginning any nutrition or exercise program. Use of the programs, advice, and information contained in this book is at the sole choice and risk of the reader.

Printed in Poland
by Amazon Fulfillment
Poland Sp. z o.o., Wrocław